SUPER EASY

DR. SEBI ALKALINE AND ANTI-INFLAMMATORY Cookbook

Quick & Easy Recipes to Reduce Inflammation, Detox Your Body, and Achieve Optimal Health | 28-Day Detox Plan Included

Kayla Rowe

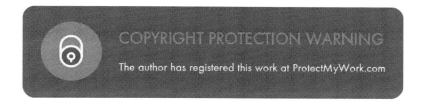

Table of Contents

INTRODUCTION

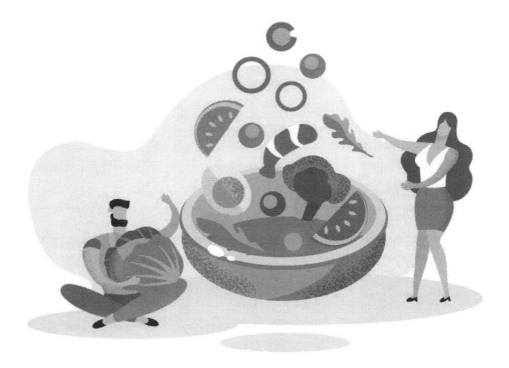

Embark on a transformative journey with a diet that reshapes how you view food and wellness, focusing on Dr. Sebi's alkaline and anti-inflammatory principles. Chronic inflammation is more than just a symptom; it's a persistent condition that can lead to severe health issues when uncontrolled. This book leverages the natural anti-inflammatory powers of foods rich in antioxidants, phytonutrients, and Omega-3 fatty acids to combat this silent threat.

By understanding the link between diet and inflammation, you'll learn how specific foods can either provoke or prevent inflammation in the body. Beyond just theoretical knowledge, the book offers practical guidance on transitioning from your current eating habits to a lifestyle abundant in healing foods, with actionable tips on pantry overhaul, smart shopping for anti-inflammatory ingredients, and meal planning strategies.

Inspired by Dr. Sebi's teachings, you'll see how simple it is to incorporate his alkaline diet principles into everyday cooking, resulting in meals that not only taste good but also promote a balanced internal environment. This approach extends to developing habits that support these dietary choices long-term, including making wise food selections when dining out and staying motivated amid challenges.

From revitalizing breakfast options to satisfying dinner recipes, every meal is an opportunity to enjoy foods that foster health without sacrificing flavor. The book also covers the essentials of hydrating and indulging responsibly, ensuring a comprehensive approach to maintaining an anti-inflammatory lifestyle.

Overview of the Alkaline Diet Concept

Step into a world where your diet mirrors the vibrant diversity of a lush garden, emphasizing foods that naturally combat inflammation. This diet isn't just a regimen but a sustainable, health-promoting lifestyle grounded in the selection of whole, nutrient-rich foods that help reduce inflammation, the body's natural yet potentially harmful response to threats.

The alkaline diet focuses on an array of colorful, anti-inflammatory foods such as berries, oranges, leafy greens, bell peppers, and tomatoes; healthful fats like those from avocados, olive oil, and omega-rich fish; and fiber-packed whole grains. Integral to this diet are herbs and spices like turmeric, ginger, and garlic, celebrated not only for their ability to enhance flavor but also their longstanding medicinal properties.

The emphasis on plant-based proteins and fatty fish over red meats, which are known to increase inflammation, underscores the diet's health-centric approach. Avoiding processed foods laden with refined sugars and unhealthy fats is also crucial, as these are known to trigger inflammation.

By embracing a diet rich in diverse, healthful ingredients, you take a proactive step toward mitigating inflammation and fostering overall health, ensuring every meal contributes positively to your well-being.

Dr. Sebi's Philosophy on Health and Nutrition

Adhering to an alkaline and anti-inflammatory diet inspired by Dr. Sebi offers a plethora of health benefits that extend beyond mere dietary changes. This approach is particularly effective in reducing symptoms associated with chronic conditions such as arthritis, including significant decreases in pain and joint stiffness.

Furthermore, the diet is instrumental in enhancing heart health by promoting the intake of omega-3 fatty acids, crucial for maintaining optimal cholesterol levels and healthy blood vessels. Dr. Sebi's teachings emphasize the importance of creating an alkaline environment within the body to stave off various diseases and maintain overall vitality.

By focusing on natural, whole foods and excluding processed items, this diet not only supports physical health but also bolsters cognitive functions, potentially reducing the risks of neurodegenerative diseases like Alzheimer's. The diet's emphasis on low-calorie density and high fiber content also aids in effective weight management, making it easier to maintain a healthy weight without sacrificing satiety or nutrition.

Moreover, by prioritizing plant-based sources and lean proteins, this dietary approach not only enhances individual health but also promotes environmental sustainability. By adopting this alkaline and anti-inflammatory lifestyle, you commit to a diet that supports personal health and ecological well-being, ensuring each meal is a step towards a healthier planet and a healthier you.

CHAPTER 1

The Science of Inflammation and Nutrition

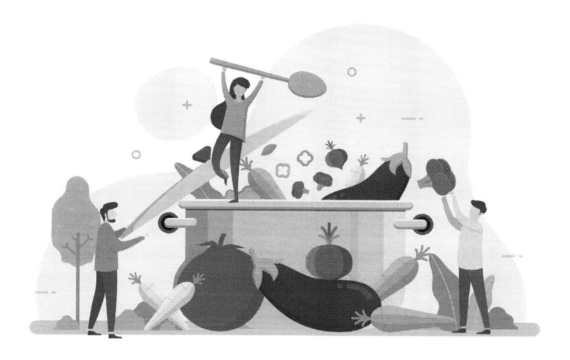

Inflammation is a term frequently mentioned in discussions about health and diet, but its implications are profound and wide-ranging. Imagine accidentally hitting your thumb with a hammer: it swells, turns red, and hurts—classic signs of acute inflammation, your body's plea for healing. Typically, inflammation is beneficial, directing your immune system to heal injuries or fend off infections. However, complications arise when the immune system malfunctions, leading to chronic inflammation—an unwelcome, persistent state of alert.

Consider inflammation as a fire alarm system. Normally, it alerts the body's "firefighters" (immune cells) to address injuries or infections. Yet, chronic inflammation is akin to a stuck alarm, continuously calling these cells to a non-existent emergency, leading to potential damage in healthy tissues. Factors like poor diet, stress, and inadequate sleep can exacerbate this condition, contributing to diseases such as rheumatoid arthritis and obesity.

Chronic inflammation is particularly perilous as it can subtly undermine health over time, contributing to serious conditions like heart disease, type 2 diabetes, and even mental health issues such as depression. It may also play a role in aging and related diseases like Alzheimer's.

Understanding these impacts underscores the importance of managing inflammation through lifestyle choices, primarily diet.

Nutritional Science Behind Anti-Inflammatory Eating

An anti-inflammatory diet focuses on whole, nutrient-dense foods that naturally counteract inflammation. Key components include fruits and vegetables rich in antioxidants and phytonutrients, such as berries, leafy greens, and citrus fruits. Omega-3 fatty acids, found in fish like salmon and plant sources like flaxseeds, play a crucial role in reducing inflammation markers. Whole grains like brown rice and quinoa, as well as spices such as turmeric and ginger, also contribute their anti-inflammatory properties.

Incorporating nuts and seeds like almonds and chia adds valuable nutrients that combat inflammation. Our recipes are designed to integrate these ingredients effectively, showing that health-focused eating can also be flavorful and satisfying. However, it's essential to understand that no single food can prevent disease. A balanced diet, regular physical activity, and stress management are fundamental to controlling inflammation.

Avoiding inflammation-promoting foods is also critical. Processed foods, sugary drinks, refined carbohydrates, and high-fat fried foods can significantly increase inflammation levels. Making gradual dietary changes, like replacing processed snacks with whole fruits or nuts, can help ease the transition to an anti-inflammatory lifestyle.

The *Role* of Antioxidants, Phytonutrients, And Omega-3s

Antioxidants are crucial in combating cellular damage caused by free radicals, unstable molecules that can deteriorate cells, accelerating aging and disease. Consuming foods high in antioxidants, such as berries, nuts, dark chocolate, and green vegetables, helps shield cells from damage and inflammation.

Phytonutrients, natural compounds found in plants, provide additional defense against threats and promote overall health. These substances are abundant in colorful fruits and vegetables and have various benefits, including anti-inflammatory properties. Regularly consuming a diverse array of produce ensures a broad intake of these beneficial compounds.

Omega-3 fatty acids are another ally against inflammation, particularly beneficial for joint health and reducing swelling and pain. Found in certain fish and plant sources, omega-3s also support heart and brain health, contributing to lower triglyceride levels and improved cognitive functions.

Incorporating a diet rich in antioxidants, phytonutrients, and omega-3s offers comprehensive support against inflammation, fostering overall wellness and disease prevention. This holistic approach to diet can profoundly influence long-term health outcomes, emphasizing the power of nutrition in maintaining bodily health and functionality.

CHAPTER 2

Transitioning to an Anti-Inflammatory Diet

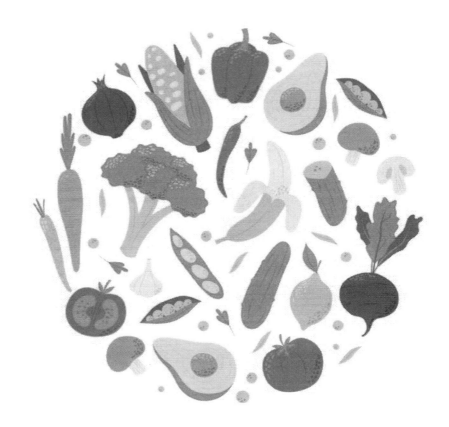

Switching to an anti-inflammatory diet involves more than just restocking your pantry; it necessitates a change in mindset. This diet is not a quick fix but a long-term commitment to enhancing your health. Processed foods, sugars, and certain dairy products can trigger chronic inflammation, leading to long-lasting health issues. In contrast, a diet rich in vegetables, fruits, lean proteins, and whole grains bolsters your body's defenses and promotes well-being.

Begin with mental preparation. Set realistic expectations and understand that results might not be immediate—wellness is a lifelong pursuit. Define clear goals, whether it's reducing symptoms of a chronic illness or boosting your energy levels, to keep yourself motivated. Educate yourself about which foods to favor and which to avoid, and familiarize yourself with meal planning and suitable recipes to ease the transition.

Anticipate challenges, such as temptations or unforeseen social events, and plan strategies to stay on track without compromising your dietary goals. Cultivate a positive outlook, viewing this change as an act of self-care and an investment in your health and happiness.

Strategies for Overcoming Old Habits:

1. **Meal Planning:** Prepare a weekly menu in advance to avoid impulsive, unhealthy eating choices.

2. **Recipe Adaptation:** Adjust your favorite recipes to include anti-inflammatory ingredients.

3. **Simplicity:** Focus on simple, nourishing meals rather than complex recipes.

4. **Support Network:** Engage with friends or family who support your dietary changes, or even better, those willing to join you in this lifestyle shift.

Physical Preparations:

- **Pantry Overhaul:** Remove inflammatory items like white bread and pastries; stock up on anti-inflammatory staples such as quinoa and brown rice.

- **Smart Shopping:** Craft a shopping list based on your meal plans, emphasizing fresh produce and whole foods.

- **Kitchen Essentials:** Ensure you have basic cooking tools like a quality knife, cutting boards, and a blender for antioxidant-rich smoothies.

- **Cooking Approach:** Start with simple recipes, such as steamed vegetables seasoned with herbs, to find enjoyment in the flavors of natural, wholesome food.

Embracing a new eating style can be challenging, and patience is crucial. Recognize that some days will be easier than others, and that resilience is key in maintaining a healthy lifestyle through all ups and downs. Each step taken, no matter how small, is a stride toward long-term health and vitality.

Pantry Cleaning – What to Discard

It's crucial to start your journey towards an anti-inflammatory diet by decluttering your pantry. Let's make room for health-promoting foods by removing those that may increase inflammation. Begin by checking the expiration dates on all packages—outdated items can lose nutritional value and even become harmful.

Here's what to look out for and remove:

1. **Refined Grains:** Products like white flour and white rice have been processed to remove fiber and essential nutrients, leading to rapid spikes in blood sugar that can provoke inflammatory responses.

2. **Sugary Snacks:** Cookies, candies, and sweetened cereals are high in added sugars, which are known contributors to inflammation.

3. **Processed Foods:** Many pre-packaged meals and snacks contain preservatives and additives that are not suited for an anti-inflammatory diet. They often include excessive sodium and unhealthy fats as well.

4. **Vegetable Oils:** Oils such as corn, safflower, and sunflower are high in omega-6 fatty acids. While essential, an imbalance of omega-6 over omega-3 fatty acids can lead to increased inflammation.

5. **Alcohol:** Regular consumption of alcohol can elevate inflammatory markers in the body, so it's important to monitor intake.

Here's a quick reference table to simplify what to discard:

Category	Examples
Refined Grains	White flour, white rice
Sugary Snacks	Cookies, candies, sweetened cereals
Processed Foods	Pre-packaged meals, snacks with additives
Vegetable Oils	Corn oil, safflower oil
Alcohol	All alcoholic beverages

Consider donating unopened and unexpired items to local food banks or shelters, reducing waste while supporting your community.

Replacing Discarded Items:

Once you've cleared out these products, replace them with healthier alternatives:

- **Whole Grains:** Stock up on quinoa, brown rice, and oatmeal.

- **Natural Sweeteners:** Use moderate amounts of honey or maple syrup if needed.

- **Healthy Fats:** Opt for extra-virgin olive oil or avocado oil.

- **Anti-inflammatory Herbs & Spices:** Incorporate turmeric, ginger, and garlic for both flavor and health benefits.

- **Nuts & Seeds:** Include sources of omega-3s like walnuts and chia seeds.

Regularly revisit your pantry every few months to keep it aligned with your health goals. A well-stocked kitchen is the foundation of good nutrition and a successful anti-inflammatory diet.

Smart Shopping for Anti-Inflammatory Foods

When shopping for anti-inflammatory foods, envision your cart as a tool for enhancing health and well-being. Each item you select plays a role in promoting an anti-inflammatory lifestyle. Here's how to make informed choices:

Vegetables: Aim for a colorful array of vegetables, as each color represents unique anti-inflammatory compounds. Opt for leafy greens like spinach, kale, and Swiss chard, which are loaded with vitamins and minerals that aid in reducing inflammation. Don't overlook cruciferous vegetables like broccoli and Brussels sprouts, which are packed with antioxidants that boost the immune system.

Fruits: Select fruits that are high in anti-inflammatory properties. Berries, such as strawberries, blueberries, raspberries, and blackberries, are rich in flavonoids. Cherries and oranges also contribute beneficial effects, primarily due to their high vitamin C content. Choose fresh or frozen fruits to ensure you get the maximum benefits.

Carbohydrates: Choose whole grains over refined ones. Grains like oats, brown rice, quinoa, and barley are better options because they contain more fiber and nutrients, which help regulate blood sugar levels and reduce inflammation.

Proteins: Include fatty fish like salmon, mackerel, sardines, and anchovies in your diet, as they are high in omega-3 fatty acids known for their anti-inflammatory effects. Plant-based proteins such as lentils, chickpeas, and beans are also excellent choices, offering additional fiber beneficial for gut health.

Dairy and Alternatives: In the dairy section, look for products containing probiotics, such as Greek yogurt and kefir, which support gut health and help control inflammation. For those avoiding dairy, choose fortified non-dairy alternatives like almond milk or soy milk.

Nuts and Seeds: Don't forget to include nuts and seeds such as almonds, walnuts, chia seeds, flaxseeds, and hemp seeds. These are rich in healthy fats and nutrients that help combat inflammation.

Fats and Oils: When selecting oils for cooking or dressings, opt for extra-virgin olive oil, which contains oleocanthal, an anti-inflammatory compound. Avocado oil is another good choice, known for its health benefits.

Herbs and Spices: Incorporate herbs and spices like turmeric and ginger into your diet. Turmeric contains curcumin, a potent anti-inflammatory compound. To enhance the absorption of curcumin, combine turmeric with black pepper.

To simplify your shopping, here's a quick reference table of anti-inflammatory essentials:

Category	Items
Vegetables	Spinach, kale, Swiss chard, broccoli, Brussels sprouts
Fruits	Berries, cherries, oranges
Carbohydrates	Oats, brown rice, quinoa, barley
Proteins	Salmon, mackerel, lentils, chickpeas
Dairy & Alternatives	Greek yogurt, kefir, almond milk
Nuts & Seeds	Almonds, walnuts, chia seeds, flaxseeds
Fats & Oils	Extra-virgin olive oil, avocado oil
Herbs & Spices	Turmeric (with black pepper), ginger

Keep this list handy, whether on your fridge or as a mobile reminder, to make smart, anti-inflammatory choices easily. This guide will help streamline your shopping experience and ensure that your diet supports your health goals effectively.

Meal Planning and Preparation Tips

Managing an anti-inflammatory diet efficiently starts with good planning and simple preparation techniques. By planning your meals, you ensure they are balanced and rich in anti-inflammatory properties. Here's how to integrate these principles seamlessly into your daily routine:

1. Meal Planning: Begin by outlining your meals for the week—breakfast, lunch, dinner, and snacks. You can write this down on paper or use a meal planning app. Ensure your meals include plenty of fruits, vegetables, whole grains, and lean proteins, and are low in processed foods, sugars, and saturated fats.

2. Shopping List Creation: Based on your meal plan, compile a shopping list. This focused approach helps avoid unnecessary purchases that can lead to both food waste and temptation. When shopping, try to stick to the store's perimeter where fresh produce and whole foods are typically located, avoiding the central aisles where processed foods prevail.

3. Meal Preparation: Set aside a few hours each week to prep your meals. This could involve washing and chopping vegetables, cooking grains like quinoa or brown rice in bulk, or preparing proteins such as grilling chicken or portioning fish. Store these prepped items in containers in your refrigerator or freezer for easy access during the week.

4. Embrace Spices: Incorporate a variety of spices—turmeric, ginger, garlic, and cinnamon— are not just flavorful, but they also boast anti-inflammatory benefits. Use these spices to enhance your meals without the need for heavy sauces or excess salt.

5. Batch Cooking: Consider cooking larger quantities of certain dishes, which can save time and energy. A large pot of vegetable stew or chili, for example, can provide several meals throughout the week or be frozen for future use.

6. Smart Snacking: Prepare healthy snacks in advance, such as vegetables with hummus, fresh fruit with nuts, or yogurt topped with berries. These quick and nutritious options will support your diet and are easy to grab on the go.

7. Stay Hydrated: Keeping hydrated is crucial in an anti-inflammatory lifestyle. Carry a reusable water bottle to encourage regular water intake throughout the day.

8. Be Flexible: Remember, flexibility is key. Life can be unpredictable, and occasionally you might need to swap meals or indulge in a treat outside your planned diet. Don't stress over these small deviations, as the overall consistency is what matters most.

By implementing these meal planning and preparation strategies, you can make your anti-inflammatory diet both manageable and enjoyable. This proactive approach helps minimize daily decision-making about food and keeps you aligned with your health goals, simplifying your lifestyle while promoting long-term well-being.

CHAPTER 3

Dr. Sebi's Alkaline Approach to an Anti-Inflammatory Diet

Navigating the myriad dietary advice available can be daunting, but Dr. Sebi's alkaline approach offers a clear and distinct path to wellness. Dr. Sebi, a renowned herbalist and healer, championed the alkaline diet as a means to restore and maintain health by reducing the body's acidity, which he linked to disease progression, including inflammation.

Key Components of Dr. Sebi's Alkaline Diet:

1. **Alkaline-rich Foods:** The diet emphasizes consuming a variety of fruits, vegetables, nuts, and selected ancient grains that promote an alkaline environment in the body.

2. **Natural Plant-Based Items:** It strictly avoids all animal products and processed foods to maintain purity and naturalness in the diet.

3. **Herbal Supplements:** Herbs are incorporated for their nutritional and therapeutic benefits, complementing the diet's healing properties.

4. **Consistent Hydration:** Dr. Sebi recommended drinking ample amounts of water, particularly alkaline or spring water, to support the body's natural detox processes.

Dr. Sebi believed that this diet would help eliminate toxins, replenish essential minerals, and enhance vitality by aligning the body with the earth's natural food sources. While traditional anti-inflammatory diets often overlap with Dr. Sebi's in their endorsement of whole foods and vegetables, there are significant differences:

- **Animal Products:** Traditional diets might include animal-based foods, especially fatty fish rich in omega-3 fatty acids, known for their anti-inflammatory properties. Dr. Sebi's diet, however, is strictly plant-based.

- **Grain Choices:** While typical anti-inflammatory diets encourage the consumption of whole grains, Dr. Sebi specifically recommends ancient grains like amaranth, which he considers more beneficial.

Comparative Table of Diet Components:

Dietary Aspect	Dr. Sebi's Alkaline Diet	Traditional Anti-Inflammatory Diet
Core Foods	Alkaline fruits, vegetables, selected nuts, and ancient grains	Whole fruits, vegetables, nuts, and whole grains
Protein Sources	Plant-based proteins only (e.g., legumes, nuts)	Includes both plant-based and animal-based proteins (e.g., fish)
Dairy and Processed Foods	Completely avoided	Limited, with some allowances depending on the specific diet
Herbal Supplements	Strong emphasis on herbal nutrition	Occasionally recommended, not as central
Water Intake	Alkaline or spring water preferred	Encouraged, type less specified

Embracing Dr. Sebi's approach to an anti-inflammatory diet involves not just following these guidelines but understanding the rationale behind each food choice. While not every aspect of his diet may suit everyone universally, beginning with a solid knowledge base allows for informed decisions about what might work best for your individual health needs. This knowledge empowers personal choice and can guide you towards a healthier, more harmonious lifestyle.

Adapting Dr. Sebi's Alkaline Regime into Your Cooking

Transitioning to Dr. Sebi's alkaline diet in your kitchen offers a promising path to enhanced health and well-being, blending nature's bounty into meals without sacrificing taste or enjoyment. Here's how you can incorporate this healthful approach into your daily cooking:

1. **Revise Your Grocery List**: Begin by modifying your shopping habits. Prioritize organic produce to minimize chemical exposure, which helps maintain an alkaline state in your body. Include a variety of whole foods such as apples, bananas, dates, berries, kale, mushrooms, cucumbers, spinach, walnuts, sesame seeds, quinoa, and rye.

2. **Eliminate Dairy and Meat**: Dr. Sebi's diet excludes dairy and meat due to their acid-forming properties. Explore plant-based alternatives like almond milk or coconut yogurt to add richness and creaminess to your dishes.

3. **Optimize Cooking Methods**: Preserve the nutrients and natural alkaline state of foods by steaming vegetables instead of boiling. Opt for baking or air-frying as healthier alternatives to deep-frying, reducing oil intake and still achieving delicious textures.

4. **Explore Exciting Substitutions**: Make your cooking an adventure with smart substitutions. Replace table salt with sea salt or Himalayan pink salt, which include beneficial trace minerals. Swap refined sugars with natural sweeteners like agave syrup or date sugar to avoid spikes in blood sugar.

5. **Flavor Without Compromise**: Utilize herbs and spices to enhance the flavors of your dishes without adding acidity. Ginger can boost digestion, turic reduces inflammation, and basil enhances immunity.

6. **Embrace Fermentation**: Incorporate fermented foods such as raw sauerkraut and kimchi into your diet. These foods introduce beneficial bacteria into your gut, aiding digestion and contributing to a healthier internal pH balance.

7. **Stay Hydrated**: Dr. Sebi emphasizes the importance of hydration. Ensure you drink plenty of water, ideally alkaline or spring water, to support the maintenance of an alkaline body.

Recipe Adaptation Example: Alkaline-Friendly Spaghetti Bolognese

- **Pasta**: Use spelt spaghetti instead of traditional wheat pasta due to its less acidic nature.

- **Base**: Replace beef mince with finely chopped mushrooms sautéed with onions, which provide a rich, savory flavor.

- **Cooking Oil**: Use grapeseed oil, which is lower in acidity compared to traditional cooking oils.

- **Sauce**: Opt for homemade tomato sauce to avoid preservatives and additives.

- **Garnish**: Enhance with fresh herbs like parsley or oregano to add flavor and nutritional benefits.

By integrating these changes, you not only adhere to an alkaline diet but also enrich your meals with health-promoting ingredients, making each dish both nourishing and enjoyable. These steps will help you maintain a healthier lifestyle in line with Dr. Sebi's teachings.

CHAPTER 4

Maintaining the Anti-Inflammatory Lifestyle

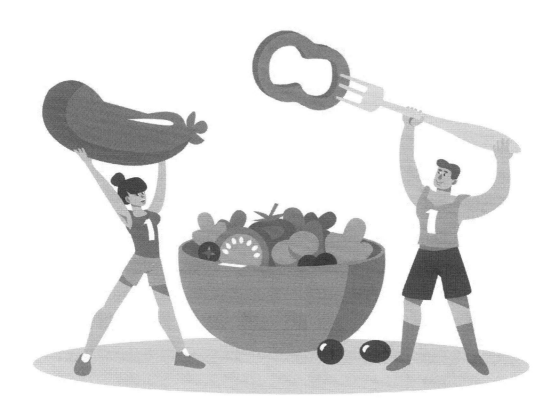

Dining Out – Making Informed Choices

Dining out can be a delightful break from the kitchen, yet it poses certain challenges when you're committed to an anti-inflammatory diet. Here's how to navigate eating out while sticking to your dietary goals:

1. **Research Restaurants Ahead of Time:** Use the internet to your advantage by checking menus online before you visit. Identify restaurants that offer dishes aligning with an anti-inflammatory diet, focusing on options that are rich in fruits, vegetables, whole grains, and lean proteins.

2. **Communicate with Your Server:** Upon arriving, don't hesitate to ask your server about the freshness of ingredients and whether dishes are made to order. Most restaurants are

willing to accommodate special requests, such as grilling rather than frying or omitting inflammatory ingredients like sugar or butter.

3. **Choosing Appetizers Wisely:** Avoid fried foods and creamy dips which are typically high in unhealthy fats. Opt for a vibrant salad loaded with leafy greens, colorful vegetables, and nuts or seeds. Request dressing on the side to better manage your intake.

4. **Select Balanced Main Courses:** Seek out dishes that provide a good balance of vegetables and protein. Choose cooking methods that retain nutritional value without adding excess fat, such as grilling or steaming. Customize your order to swap out deep-fried sides with steamed vegetables or a side salad.

5. **Prefer Whole Grains:** For dishes involving pasta or bread, go for whole grain options. These offer more fiber and nutrients than refined grains. If available, brown rice or quinoa are excellent choices that are not only healthier but also satisfying.

6. **Opt for Beneficial Proteins:** Favor protein sources like salmon, mackerel, or trout, which are rich in omega-3 fatty acids and known for their anti-inflammatory effects. If you prefer other meats, select lean cuts such as sirloin or skinless poultry to minimize saturated fat consumption.

7. **Make Smart Beverage Choices:** Hydration is key, but avoid sugary drinks as they can exacerbate inflammation. Choose water, herbal teas, or green tea, which are rich in antioxidants. If you enjoy alcohol, red wine is a better option in moderation, thanks to its resveratrol content.

8. **Dessert Choices:** Opt for desserts that align with your diet, such as fresh fruits which satisfy the sweet tooth without adding processed sugars. These choices are delicious and packed with beneficial nutrients.

9. **Suggesting Recipes to Chefs:** If you're fond of a particular dish from this cookbook, consider suggesting it to the chef. Many chefs enjoy the challenge of crafting something new, and you'll get to enjoy your favorite meal prepared with care.

By planning ahead and communicating clearly with the restaurant staff, you can ensure that dining out complements your anti-inflammatory lifestyle, allowing you to enjoy social outings without compromising your health goals.

Sustaining Motivation Over Time

Maintaining enthusiasm for an anti-inflammatory lifestyle over the long term can be challenging, especially when progress seems slow or temptations arise frequently. This section offers strategies to keep your motivation high, ensuring your commitment to health remains strong.

1. **Set Realistic Goals:** Start by setting achievable objectives. Rather than expecting dramatic changes immediately, celebrate smaller victories, like integrating a new anti-inflammatory recipe into your diet each week. Incremental success builds sustainable habits.

2. **Use Visual Reminders:** Place a chart or table on your refrigerator door that lists "Anti-Inflammatory Foods to Enjoy" and "Foods to Avoid." This can serve as a constant, gentle reminder to make healthier choices without feeling overwhelmed.

3. **Keep an Inspiration Journal:** Document why you started this diet and any moments of inspiration. Reviewing this journal can provide a motivational boost during tougher times. Also, track your progress, noting any physical improvements, changes in inflammation markers, or weight loss. Seeing tangible results can be incredibly encouraging.

4. **Seek Community Support:** Engage with others who are following similar dietary paths. Whether through online forums, local support groups, or anti-inflammatory diet cooking classes, connecting with peers can offer encouragement and new ideas.

5. **Educate Yourself:** Continue learning about the anti-inflammatory effects of different foods and their health benefits. Understanding the "why" behind your food choices deepens your commitment and makes your dietary decisions more impactful.

6. **Be Gentle with Setbacks:** Recognize that setbacks are part of the journey. If you make a less healthy choice, don't be too hard on yourself. Remember, it's your overall pattern of eating that matters most, not occasional slips.

7. **Celebrate Milestones:** Take time to celebrate your successes, no matter how small. Whether it's a week without processed sugar or increasing the proportion of vegetables in your meals, these milestones signify substantial progress towards a healthier lifestyle.

By implementing these strategies, you can maintain your drive and commitment to an anti-inflammatory lifestyle. Each small step is part of a larger journey towards health and well-being, and recognizing your progress along the way can provide the motivation needed to continue.

Dealing With Setbacks and How to Bounce Back

Setbacks are a normal part of any journey, especially when adapting to a new dietary pattern like an anti-inflammatory diet. Whether it's a special occasion that tempts you with non-dietary foods or a stressful day that drives you toward old comfort foods, it's important to handle these moments constructively. Here's how you can bounce back and stay on track:

1. **Acknowledge the Slip:** Understand that slips are a normal part of the change process. Accepting that it happened without self-judgment is the first step to moving forward.

2. **Reflect on Triggers:** Spend some time thinking about what led to the setback. Was it emotional, situational, or simply a matter of convenience? Identifying these triggers can help you plan to avoid them in the future.

3. **Plan Ahead:** Keep ready-to-eat healthy meals or ingredients at hand to prevent impulsive, non-compliant eating. Preparation is key to staying on track.

4. **Start Fresh, Immediately:** Don't wait for a new day or week to get back on your plan. The next meal is your next chance to align with your anti-inflammatory goals.

5. **Seek Support:** Reach out to a supportive friend, family member, or a group who understands your goals. Sharing your experiences and challenges can bolster your resolve and motivation.

Bounce Back Table

Step	Action	Example
Acknowledge	Accept the slip without guilt.	"It's okay, one meal doesn't define my journey."
Reflect	Identify what led to the slip.	"It was social pressure at the party."
Plan	Prepare for future similar situations.	Keep a go-to healthy dish ready, like frozen stew.
Start Fresh	Resume the diet immediately.	Have an anti-inflammatory breakfast like oatmeal with berries and nuts.
Seek Support	Talk to someone who supports your goals.	Call a friend who also follows an anti-inflammatory diet.

Remember, setbacks are not only common but also opportunities for growth and learning. Each challenge you overcome reinforces your commitment and enhances your ability to make healthier choices. An occasional indulgence does not have to derail your efforts; with the right mindset and strategies, you can maintain your path to wellness.

Breakfast Recipes

6. Omega Boost Avocado Toast

Preparation time: Five mins

Cooking time: N/A

Servings: Two

Ingredients:

- One ripe avocado
- Two whole-grain bread slices, toasted
- One tsp lemon juice
- Half tsp ground flaxseed
- A pinch of salt & black pepper
- One tbsp chia seeds (optional)

Directions:

1. In your container, mash the ripe avocado and mix in lemon juice, ground flaxseed, salt, and pepper.

2. Divide the avocado mixture onto the toasted bread evenly. Sprinkle chia seeds on top for an extra omega boost (optional).

Serving Size: One piece of toast

Nutritional Values (per serving): Calories: 250; Carbs: 27g; Fat: 15g; Protein: 6g; Fiber: 7g

7. Sweet Potato & Red Onion Hash

Preparation time: Fifteen mins

Cooking time: Twenty-five mins

Servings: Four

Ingredients:

- Two big sweet potatoes, peeled & diced

- One big red onion, sliced

- Three tbsp olive oil

- One tsp smoked paprika

- Half tsp garlic powder

- Quarter tsp sea salt

Directions:

1. Warm up your oven to 400°F. Mix sweet potatoes and red onion on your baking sheet. Drizzle using olive oil and sprinkle paprika, garlic powder, and sea salt on top. Mix well.

2. Roast for twenty-five mins till sweet potatoes are tender. Serve.

Serving Size: One cup

Nutritional Values (per serving): Calories: 350; Carbs: 50g; Fat: 14g; Protein: 5g; Fiber: 6g

8. Anti-Inflammatory Granola Clusters

Preparation time: Ten mins

Cooking time: Twenty mins

Servings: Six

Ingredients:

- Two cups rolled oats

- One cup raw almonds, chopped

- Two tbsp chia seeds

- Half tsp ground cinnamon

- Quarter tsp sea salt

- Quarter cup honey

- Three tbsp coconut oil, melted

Directions:

1. Warm up your oven to 350°F. In your big container, mix oats, almonds, chia seeds, cinnamon, and sea salt. Add honey and coconut oil, then mix well till clusters form.

2. Spread the mixture evenly on your lined baking sheet. Bake for twenty mins till golden brown.

3. Let it cool completely as it will become crunchier as it cools down. Break granola into clusters, then store or serve.

Serving Size: One-third of a cup

Nutritional Values (per serving): Calories: 280; Carbs: 32g; Fat: 16g; Protein: 7g; Fiber: 5g

9. *Turmeric Ginger Oatmeal*

Preparation time: Five mins

Cooking time: Five mins

Servings: Two

Ingredients:

- One cup rolled oats

- Two cups almond milk or water

- One tbsp turmeric powder

- Half tbsp ginger, grated

- One tsp cinnamon powder

- One tsp honey or maple syrup (optional)

- A pinch of salt

Directions:

1. In your saucepan on moderate temp, let almond milk boil. Add rolled oats, then adjust to a simmer.

2. Mix in turmeric powder, grated ginger, cinnamon powder, and salt. Continue to simmer for five mins till oats are cooked. Drizzle with honey for sweetness if desired.

Serving Size: Half a cup cooked oatmeal

Nutritional Values (per serving): Calories: 172; Carbs: 29g; Fat: 3g; Protein: 4g; Fiber: 4g

10. Blueberry Spinach Smoothie Bowl

Preparation time: Five mins

Cooking time: N/A

Servings: Two

Ingredients:

- One cup fresh blueberries

- Two cups fresh baby spinach

- One tbsp chia seeds

- One & half cups unsweetened almond milk

- One tbsp raw honey

- Half tsp ground cinnamon

- One tbsp almond butter

Directions:

1. Mix blueberries, spinach, almond milk, chia seeds, honey, cinnamon, and almond butter in your high-speed blender.

2. Blend on high till smooth. Pour into two bowls, then serve.

Serving Size: Half the prepared amount

Nutritional Values (per serving): Calories 150; Carbs 18g; Fat 7g; Protein 5g; Fiber 4g

11. Chia Seed & Mixed Berry Parfait

Preparation time: Ten mins

Cooking time: N/A

Servings: Two

Ingredients:

- Three tbsp chia seeds

- One cup unsweetened coconut milk

- One cup mixed berries

- Half cup Greek yogurt

- One tbsp honey

- Quarter tsp vanilla extract

Directions:

1. In your container, mix chia seeds and coconut milk. Cover and refrigerate for at least ten mins.

2. In serving glasses, create layers by adding half of the gelled chia mixture into each glass. Add a layer of mixed berries over the chia layer.

3. Top with Greek yogurt, drizzle with honey or maple syrup, and add vanilla extract. Repeat the layers if desired. Serve.

Serving Size: Half the prepared amount

Nutritional Values (per serving): Calories 200; Carbs 24g; Fat 9g; Protein 8g; Fiber 10g

12. Quinoa & Almond Breakfast Bars

Preparation time: Fifteen mins

Cooking time: Twenty-five mins

Servings: Six

Ingredients:

- One cup cooked quinoa

- Three tbsp honey

- Two tbsp coconut oil, melted

- Half cup almonds, chopped

- One cup rolled oats

- One tsp cinnamon

- A pinch of salt

Directions:

1. Warm up your oven to 350°F. In your big container, mix cooked quinoa, honey, coconut oil, almonds, oats, cinnamon, and salt.

2. Press the quinoa mixture firmly into your lined eight-inch square baking dish. Bake for twenty-five mins till the bars are golden brown. Cool it down, then slice into six bars. Serve.

Serving Size: One bar

Nutritional Values (per serving): Calories: 250; Carbs: 32g; Fat: 10g; Protein: 6g; Fiber: 4g

13. *Kale and Mushroom Frittata*

Preparation time: Ten mins

Cooking time: Twenty mins

Servings: Four

Ingredients:

- Four cups kale, stems removed & leaves chopped

- One cup sliced mushrooms

- Six big eggs, beaten

- Two tbsp olive oil

- One tsp garlic powder

- Salt & pepper, as required

- Quarter cup almond milk

Directions:

1. Warm up your oven to 375°F.

2. In your ovenproof skillet on moderate temp, warm up oil, then sauté kale and mushrooms with garlic powder, salt, and pepper for five mins.

3. Pour the beaten eggs mixed with almond milk. Cook without stirring for three mins.

4. Transfer skillet to your oven and bake for fifteen mins till eggs are set. Slice into four pieces and serve.

Serving Size: One quarter of frittata

Nutritional Values (per serving): Calories: 180; Carbs: 5g; Fat: 12g; Protein: 14g; Fiber: 2g

14. Green Tea Infused Chia Pudding

Preparation time: Fifteen mins

Cooking time: N/A

Servings: Four

Ingredients:

- Three tbsp chia seeds
- One cup unsweetened almond milk
- One tbsp pure maple syrup
- Half tsp vanilla extract
- One tbsp matcha green tea powder
- Fresh mixed berries for topping

Directions:

1. In your medium-sized container, whisk almond milk, maple syrup, vanilla, and matcha green tea powder. Add chia seeds, then mix for one minute.

2. Let the mixture sit for five mins, then stir again. Cover, then refrigerate for at least four hours. Serve in individual bowls and top with berries.

Serving Size: Half cup

Nutritional Values (per serving): Calories; 120; Carbs; 15g; Fat; 5g; Protein; 4g; Fiber 5g

15. Broccoli and Bell Pepper Mini Quiche

Preparation time: Twenty mins

Cooking time: Twenty-five mins

Servings: Six

Ingredients:

Four eggs

- One cup chopped broccoli florets

- Half cup diced red bell peppers

- One cup shredded zucchini (excess water removed)

- Quarter cup almond milk

- Half tsp garlic powder

- Quarter tsp turmeric powder

Directions:

1. Warm up your oven to 350°F, then lightly grease your six-cup muffin pan. In your big container, whisk eggs, almond milk, garlic powder, and turmeric till smooth.

2. Mix in broccoli, bell peppers, and zucchini till well combined. Divide it among your muffin cups.

3. Bake for twenty to twenty-five mins till the mini quiches are firm. Cool them down, then serve.

Serving Size: One mini quiche

Nutritional Values (per serving): Calories; 90; Carbs; 4g; Fat; 6g; Protein; 7g; Fiber 1g

16. Flaxseed and Walnut Porridge

Preparation time: Five mins

Cooking time: Ten mins

Servings: Two

Ingredients:

- One cup unsweetened almond milk

- Quarter cup flaxseeds

- Half cup chopped walnuts

- One tbsp honey

- One tbsp cinnamon

- Salt, as required

Directions:

1. In your small saucepan, let almond milk simmer on moderate temp. Add flaxseeds, mix well, then cook for five mins till it begins to thicken.

2. Mix in the cinnamon and salt. Remove, then let it sit for five mins to thicken further. Serve warm garnished with walnuts and drizzle with honey.

Serving Size: One bowl

Nutritional Values (per serving): Calories 280; Carbs 18g; Fat 22g; Protein 8g; Fiber 9g

17. Cauliflower Rice Breakfast Bowl

Preparation time: Ten mins

Cooking time: Ten mins

Servings: Two

Ingredients:

- Four cups cauliflower rice
- Two tbsp olive oil
- Four big eggs
- One tbsp lemon juice
- Two tbsp fresh parsley, chopped
- Salt & black pepper, as required

Directions:

1. In your big skillet on moderate temp, warm up oil, then cook cauliflower rice with salt and pepper for seven mins till soft.

2. In another pan, cook eggs to your liking—poached or sunny-side up works well.

3. Divide the cauliflower rice into bowls, top each with two eggs, sprinkle with parsley, then drizzle with lemon juice. Serve.

Serving Size: One bowl

Nutritional Values (per serving): Calories 320; Carbs 14g; Fat 24g; Protein 18g; Fiber 5g

18. Anti-Oxidant Rich Buckwheat Pancakes

Preparation time: Ten mins

Cooking time: Fifteen mins

Servings: Four

Ingredients:

- One & half cups buckwheat flour
- One tbsp ground flaxseed
- Two tsp baking powder
- Half tsp ground cinnamon
- One cup unsweetened almond milk
- One big egg
- Two tbsp pure maple syrup

Directions:

1. In your big container, whisk buckwheat flour, flaxseed, baking powder, and cinnamon.
2. In another container, beat almond milk, egg, and maple syrup. Combine it with flour mixture till blended.
3. Warm up your non-stick skillet on moderate temp and scoop Quarter-cup batter for each pancake.
4. Cook for two to three mins on one side, then flip and cook for two mins till golden. Serve.

Serving Size: Two pancakes

Nutritional Values (per serving): Calories 250; Carbs 45g; Fat 5g; Protein 10g; Fiber 8g

19. Apple Cinnamon Overnight Oats

Preparation time: Five mins + chilling time

Cooking time: N/A

Servings: Two

Ingredients:

- One cup rolled oats

- One tbsp chia seeds

- One cup unsweetened almond milk

- Half cup diced apple

- One tsp ground cinnamon

- One tbsp pure maple syrup

- Salt, as required

Directions:

1. In your mason jar or container, mix rolled oats and chia seeds. Add almond milk, apple, cinnamon, maple syrup, and salt. Mix well. Cover, then refrigerate overnight.

2. In the morning, mix oats and add a little more almond milk if desired. Serve cold.

Serving Size: Half of the prepared mixture

Nutritional Values (per serving): Calories 315; Carbs 55g; Fat 7g; Protein 8g; Fiber 10g

20. Spinach and Tomato Omelette

Preparation time: Five mins

Cooking time: Ten mins

Servings: Two

Ingredients:

- Four big eggs

- One cup fresh spinach, chopped

- One medium tomato, diced

- Two tbsp olive oil

- Quarter tsp salt

- Quarter tsp black pepper

Directions:

1. In your container, whisk eggs till well beaten. Mix in spinach and tomato.

2. Warm up oil in your non-stick pan on moderate temp. Pour egg mixture into it, tilting to spread evenly.

3. Cook for five mins, then flip and cook for five mins. Flavor it using salt and pepper. Serve.

Serving Size: Half of the omelette

Nutritional Values (per serving): Calories 250; Carbs 6g; Fat 18g; Protein 14g; Fiber 2g

Lunch Recipes

21. Stuffed Bell Peppers with Spinach

Preparation time: Ten mins

Cooking time: Twenty-five mins

Servings: Four

Ingredients:

- Four medium bell peppers, tops cut off and seeded

- One cup quinoa, cooked

- One cup spinach leaves, chopped

- One cup cherry tomatoes, halved

- Two tbsp olive oil

- Half tsp garlic powder

- Quarter tsp salt

Directions:

1. Warm up your oven to 375°F. In your container, mix quinoa, spinach, cherry tomatoes, garlic powder, salt, and one tbsp oil.

2. Stuff each bell pepper with it, then put in your baking dish. Drizzle remaining olive oil on top.

3. Bake for twenty-five mins till peppers are tender. Serve.

Serving Size: One stuffed pepper

Nutritional Values (per serving): Calories 180; Carbs 27g; Fat 7g; Protein 6g; Fiber 5g

22. Tomatoes and Bell Pepper Gazpacho

Preparation time: Fifteen mins

Cooking time: N/A

Servings: Four

Ingredients:

- Four cups ripe tomatoes, chopped

- One cup red bell pepper, chopped

- One cucumber, peeled and chopped

- Two tbsp red onion, minced

- One tbsp apple cider vinegar

- Three tbsp olive oil

- Quarter tsp sea salt

Directions:

1. Mix tomatoes, bell pepper, cucumber, and red onion in your big container.

2. In your blender, blend your mixture till smooth. Transfer it back into your bowl, then mix in apple cider, oil, and sea salt. Chill in your refrigerator, then serve.

Serving Size: One cup

Nutritional Values (per serving): Calories: 123; Carbs: 14g; Fat: 7g; Protein: 2g; Fiber: 3g

23. Sweet Potato and Lentil Stew

Preparation time: Twenty mins

Cooking time: Twenty-five mins

Servings: Four servings

Ingredients:

- One-lb. sweet potatoes, peeled & cubed

- Three-fourths cup dry green lentils

- One tbsp olive oil

- One tsp ground turmeric

- Five cups vegetable broth

- Two minced cloves garlic

- Sea salt, as required

Directions:

1. Warm up oil on moderate temp in your big pot, then sauté garlic till fragrant. Add sweet potatoes, lentils, turmeric, and broth.

2. Let it boil, then adjust to a simmer for twenty-five mins till lentils are cooked. Flavor it using sea salt, then serve.

Serving Size: One & half cups

Nutritional Values (per serving): Calories: 250; Carbs: 38g; Fat: 5g; Protein: 12g; Fiber: 15g

24. *Turmeric-Ginger Grilled Chicken*

Preparation time: Fifteen mins

Cooking time: Twenty-five mins

Servings: Four

Ingredients:

- Four chicken breasts, boneless and skinless

- One tbsp olive oil

- Two tsp turmeric powder

- Two tsp ginger, grated

- One tsp garlic powder

- Half tsp black pepper

- One lemon (juice for marinade)

Directions:

1. In your container, whisk oil, turmeric powder, ginger, garlic powder, pepper, and lemon juice. Coat chicken breasts with it, then let it sit for fifteen mins.

2. Warm up your grill to moderate-high temp. Grill chicken breasts for twelve mins per side till internal temperature reaches one hundred sixty-five degrees Fahrenheit.

Serving Size: One grilled chicken breast

Nutritional Values (per serving): Calories: 300; Carbs: 2g; Fat: 13g; Protein: 46g; Fiber: 1g

25. *Wild Salmon and Roasted Veggie Bowl*

Preparation time: Fifteen mins

Cooking time: Twenty-five mins

Servings: Four

Ingredients:

- Four (six-ounce) wild salmon fillets

- Two cups broccoli florets

- One cup cherry tomatoes, halved

- Quarter cup red onion slices

- Two tbsp olive oil

- Half tsp sea salt

- One tsp ground black pepper

Directions:

1. Warm up your oven to 400°F. On your baking sheet, toss broccoli, cherry tomatoes, and onion with oil, sea salt, and pepper.

2. Roast vegetables for fifteen mins. Remove your tray, then create space to put salmon fillets among your vegetables.

3. Return to your oven and bake for ten mins till salmon is cooked through. Serve.

Serving Size: One bowl

Nutritional Values (per serving): Calories 345; Carbs 9g; Fat 19g; Protein 34g; Fiber 3g

26. *Turkey, Spinach, and Cucumber Wrap*

Preparation time: Fifteen mins

Cooking time: N/A

Servings: Four

Ingredients:

- Four big whole-grain tortillas

- One lb. sliced turkey breast

- Two cups fresh spinach leaves

- One medium cucumber, thinly sliced

- Four tbsp hummus

- One tsp dried Italian herbs

Directions:

1. Lay out your tortillas, then spread one tbsp hummus on each. Evenly distribute the turkey slices over the hummus.

2. Top with spinach and cucumber, then sprinkle Italian herbs. Roll up your tortillas tightly and cut in half.

Serving Size: One wrap

Nutritional Values (per serving): Calories: 320; Carbs: 36g; Fat: 9g; Protein: 24g; Fiber: 5g

27. Quick Broccoli Almond Soup

Preparation time: Fifteen mins

Cooking time: Twenty-five mins

Servings: Four

Ingredients:

- Four cups broccoli florets

- Two cups low-sodium vegetable broth

- One cup unsweetened almond milk

- One tbsp olive oil

- One tsp minced garlic

- One-fourth cup raw almonds, chopped

- Half tsp sea salt

Directions:

1. In your big pot, warm up oil on moderate temp. Add garlic, then cook for one minute till fragrant. Add broccoli and sea salt, then cook for three mins.

2. Pour in broth and almond milk, then let it boil. Adjust to a simmer for twenty mins till the broccoli is tender.

3. Puree soup using your immersion blender till smooth. Top it with almonds, then serve.

Serving Size: One cup

Nutritional Values (per serving): Calories: 150; Carbs: 11g; Fat: 10g; Protein: 6g; Fiber: 4g

28. *Berry Walnut Baby Spinach Salad*

Preparation time: Ten mins

Cooking time: N/A

Servings: Two

Ingredients:

- Four cups baby spinach

- One cup mixed berries

- Quarter cup walnuts, roughly chopped

- Two tbsp of balsamic vinegar

- One tbsp olive oil

- Salt, as required

Directions:

1. In your big container, toss baby spinach with berries and walnuts.

2. In your small container, whisk balsamic vinegar, oil, and salt. Drizzle it on your salad, then toss gently. Serve.

3. Divide the salad into two serving plates, and serve immediately for maximum freshness.

Serving Size: Half of total salad

Nutritional Values (per serving): Calories 235; Carbs 18g; Fat 16g; Protein 5g; Fiber 4g

29. Smoked Salmon and Avocado Wrap

Preparation time: Ten mins

Cooking time: N/A

Servings: Two

Ingredients:

- Two whole-grain wrap breads

- Four oz smoked salmon

- One ripe avocado, sliced thinly

- One cup arugula

- Four tbsp cream cheese (choose dairy-free if preferable)

- One tbsp lemon juice

- Black pepper, as required

Directions:

Lay out whole-grain wraps on your flat surface. Spread two tbsp cream cheese on each wrap. Put two oz smoked salmon on each wrap. Arrange avocado and arugula on salmon.

Drizzle half lemon juice, then flavor it using black pepper. Roll up your wraps tightly, cut them in half diagonally, then serve.

Serving Size: One wrap (cut in half)

Nutritional Values (per serving): Calories 380; Carbs 34g; Fat 20g; Protein 22g; Fiber 8g

30. Lemon Garlic Baked Cod with Asparagus

Preparation time: Ten mins

Cooking time: Fifteen mins

Servings: Four

Ingredients:

- Four (six-oz) cod fillets

- Two tbsp olive oil

- One tbsp lemon juice

- Three cloves minced garlic

- One lb. asparagus, trimmed

- One tsp grated lemon zest

- Half tsp sea salt

Directions:

Warm up your oven to 400°F. Arrange cod fillets and asparagus on your lined baking sheet.

In your small container, whisk oil, lemon juice, garlic, zest, and sea salt. Drizzle it on your cod and asparagus. Bake for fifteen mins till cod flakes easily. Serve.

Serving Size: One fillet with equal portion of asparagus

Nutritional Values (per serving): Calories: 220; Carbs: 7g; Fat: 9g; Protein: 29g; Fiber: 3g

31. Beetroot and Carrot Detox Salad

Preparation time: Fifteen mins

Cooking time: N/A

Servings: Four servings

Ingredients:

- Two cups grated beetroot

- Two cups grated carrot

- One tbsp olive oil

- Two tbsp lemon juice

- One tsp ground cumin

- Quarter cup chopped parsley

- Salt, as required

Directions:

1. In your big container, mix beetroot and carrot. Add oil, lemon juice, cumin, and salt. Toss to mix.

2. Sprinkle with parsley, then serve.

Serving Size: One cup

Nutritional Values (per serving): Calories: 120; Carbs: 15g; Fat: 5g; Protein: 2g; Fiber: 4g

32. Spicy Lentil and Turmeric Soup

Preparation time: Ten mins

Cooking time: Twenty-five mins

Servings: Four

Ingredients:

- One cup red lentils, washed

- Three cups vegetable broth

- One can (14 oz) diced tomatoes

- Two tsp turmeric powder

- One tsp cayenne pepper

- Two tbsp coconut oil

- Salt, as required

Directions:

1. In your pot, warm up coconut oil on moderate temp, then add turmeric and cayenne pepper, mixing for one minute. Add lentils, tomatoes, and broth.

2. Let it boil, then simmer for twenty-five mins till lentils are soft. Flavor it using salt, then serve hot.

Serving Size: One and a half cups

Nutritional Values (per serving): Calories: 215; Carbs: 30g; Fat: 7g; Protein: 12g; Fiber: 6g

33. Curried Chickpea Lettuce Wraps

Preparation time: Twenty mins

Cooking time: N/A

Servings: Four

Ingredients:

- Two cups canned chickpeas, strained & washed
- Four big lettuce leaves
- Two tbsp tahini
- One tbsp curry powder
- Half cup chopped red bell pepper
- Two tbsp chopped fresh cilantro
- One tsp fresh lime juice

Directions:

1. In your container, mash the chickpeas till coarsely crushed. Add tahini, curry powder, lime juice, red bell pepper, and cilantro. Mix well.
2. Spoon chickpea mixture into each lettuce leaf, then serve.

Serving Size: One lettuce wrap

Nutritional Values (per serving): Calories: 180; Carbs: 20g; Fat: 6g; Protein: 8g; Fiber: 6g

34. Butternut Squash and Turmeric Soup

Preparation time: Fifteen mins

Cooking time: Twenty-five mins

Servings: Four

Ingredients:

- Four cups cubed butternut squash
- One tbsp olive oil

- One tsp ground turmeric

- Half tsp black pepper

- One quart low-sodium vegetable broth

- One cup chopped onions

- Three cloves garlic, minced

Directions:

1. In your big pot on moderate temp, add oil, onions, and garlic. Sauté for five mins till the onions become translucent.

2. Add butternut squash, turmeric, black pepper, and broth. Let it boil. Adjust to a simmer for twenty mins till squash is tender.

3. Puree the soup using your immersion blender till smooth. Serve hot.

Serving Size: One and a half cups

Nutritional Values (per serving): Calories 152; Carbs 35g; Fat 2g; Protein 3g; Fiber 6g

35. *Grilled Vegetable Hummus Wrap*

Preparation time: Ten mins

Cooking time: Ten mins

Servings: Four

Ingredients:

- Four whole grain wraps

- One cup hummus

- Two red bell peppers, sliced

- Two zucchinis, thinly sliced lengthwise

- One tbsp olive oil

- Half tsp garlic powder

- Half tsp dried oregano

Directions:

1. Warm up your grill to moderate-high temp. Toss bell peppers and zucchinis with oil, garlic powder, and oregano.

2. Grill them for three mins on each side till charred. Spread quarter cup hummus on each wrap.

3. Divide grilled vegetables among wraps, then roll them up tightly. Serve.

Serving Size: One wrap

Nutritional Values (per serving): Calories 330; Carbs 45g; Fat 12g; Protein 12g; Fiber 8g

Dinner Recipes

36. Ginger-Turmeric Cauliflower Steaks

Preparation time: Fifteen mins

Cooking time: Twenty-five mins

Servings: Four servings

Ingredients:

- One big head cauliflower, discard leaves & sliced into four even steaks
- Two tbsp olive oil
- One tsp turmeric
- Half tsp ginger, freshly grated
- Quarter tsp black pepper, freshly ground
- Half tsp sea salt

Directions:

1. Warm up your oven to 400°F.
2. In your small container, mix oil with turmeric, ginger, salt, and black pepper. Brush each cauliflower steak with it.
3. Put cauliflower steaks on your baking sheet and roast for twenty-five mins, flipping once through till golden brown and tender. Serve.

Serving Size: One cauliflower steak

Nutritional Values (per serving): Calories 120; Carbs 10g; Fat 7g; Protein 3g; Fiber 4g

37. Black Bean Quinoa Casserole

Preparation time: Fifteen mins

Cooking time: Thirty mins

Servings: Four

Ingredients:

- One cup quinoa, rinsed

- Two cups water

- One can (15 oz) black beans, strained & washed

- One cup frozen corn kernels

- One cup diced tomatoes

- One tbsp chili powder

- One tsp cumin

- Salt, as required

Directions:

1. Warm up your oven to 375°F.

2. In your medium saucepan, mix quinoa and water, then let it boil. Cover, then simmer for fifteen mins, till most of the water is absorbed.

3. In your big container, mix cooked quinoa, black beans, corn, tomatoes, chili powder, cumin, and salt.

4. Transfer it to your baking dish and bake uncovered for fifteen mins. Serve.

Serving Size: One quarter of the dish

Nutritional Values (per serving): Calories 350; Carbs 60g; Fat 3g; Protein 15g; Fiber 10g

38. Garlicky Shrimp and Broccoli Rabe

Preparation time: Ten mins

Cooking time: Fifteen mins

Servings: Four

Ingredients:

- One lb. shrimp, peeled & deveined

- Two bunches broccoli rabe, trimmed & chopped

- Four tbsp olive oil

- Three cloves garlic, minced

- One tsp crushed red pepper flakes (optional)

- Salt, as required

Directions:

1. Warm up two tbsp oil in your big pan on moderate temp. Add garlic and red pepper flakes if using, then sauté for one minute till fragrant.

2. Add broccoli rabe, then cook for five mins till it is tender. Remove broccoli rabe, then put it aside on your plate.

3. In your same pan, add remaining oil and adjust to moderate-high temp. Add shrimp and cook for two to three mins per side till they are pink all over.

4. Add broccoli rabe, then toss well. Warm it through for one minute. Flavor it using salt and serve hot.

Serving Size: Six shrimp with equal parts broccoli rabe

Nutritional Values (per serving): Calories 240; Carbs 4g; Fat 10g; Protein 35g; Fiber 2g

39. Omega 3-Rich Salmon with Zucchini Ribbons

Preparation time: Fifteen mins

Cooking time: Fifteen mins

Servings: Two

Ingredients:

- Two (six-ounce) salmon fillets

- Four tsp olive oil

- One big zucchini, sliced into thin ribbons

- One tsp lemon zest

- Half tsp sea salt

- Quarter tsp black pepper, ground

- Two tbsp fresh dill, chopped

Directions:

1. Warm up your grill to moderate temp. Brush salmon fillets with two tsp oil, then flavor it using sea salt and pepper. Grill the salmon for four to five mins per side till fully cooked.

2. In the last couple of mins of cooking, add the zucchini ribbons and cook till tender-crisp. Toss the zucchini with remaining oil, zest, dill, salt and pepper.

3. Serve the salmon fillets on a bed of zucchini ribbons.

Serving Size: One fillet with half of zucchini ribbons

Nutritional Values (per serving): Calories 365; Carbs 6g; Fat 23g; Protein 34g; Fiber 2g

40. Spicy Tomato-Basil Farro with Olives

Preparation time: Ten mins

Cooking time: Thirty mins

Servings: Four

Ingredients:

- One cup farro, washed

- Two cans (fourteen oz each) of diced tomatoes

- One cup pitted Kalamata olives

- Three cloves garlic, minced

- Two tbsp fresh basil, chopped

- One tbsp olive oil

- Half tsp crushed red pepper flakes

Directions:

1. Warm up oil in your big pot on moderate temp, then cook garlic for two mins till fragrant. Add farro and toast lightly for two mins.

2. Pour tomatoes and their juice along with one and half cups water. Mix in red pepper flakes.

3. Let it boil, cover and cook for twenty-five mins till farro is tender. Remove, then stir in olives and basil before serving.

Serving Size: One-fourth of total dish

Nutritional Values (per serving): Calories 370; Carbs 50g; Fat 12g; Protein 10g; Fiber 8g

41. Balsamic Grilled Tempeh with Veggies

Preparation time: Ten mins

Cooking time: Fifteen mins

Servings: Four

Ingredients:

- Eight ounces tempeh, cut into cubes

- One tbsp balsamic vinegar

- Two tbsp olive oil

- One red bell pepper, cut into pieces

- One zucchini, sliced into half-moons

- Half lb. asparagus spears, trimmed

- One tsp garlic powder

- Quarter tsp sea salt

Directions:

1. Warm up your grill to moderate temp.

2. In your small container, whisk balsamic vinegar, olive oil, garlic powder and salt. Toss tempeh and veggies in it till coated.

3. Thread tempeh cubes and vegetables onto skewers. Grill skewers for fifteen mins, turning occasionally till tempeh is browned.

Serving Size: Two skewers

Nutritional Values (per serving): Calories 200; Carbs 13g; Fat 12g; Protein 11g; Fiber 3g

42. Citrus-Herb Baked Cod Fillets

Preparation time: Fifteen mins

Cooking time: Twenty mins

Servings: Four

Ingredients:

- Four (one pound total) cod fillets

- Two tbsp olive oil

- One tbsp fresh lemon juice

- Two tsp grated orange zest

- One tbsp chopped fresh dill

- One tsp minced garlic

- Quarter tsp sea salt

Directions:

1. Warm up your oven to 350°F. In your small container, mix oil, lemon juice, zest, dill, garlic, and sea salt to create the citrus-herb marinade.

2. Put cod fillets in your baking dish, then coat them with the marinade. Bake for twenty mins till fish flakes easily. Serve.

Serving Size: One cod fillet

Nutritional Values (per serving): Calories 190; Carbs 1g; Fat 7g; Protein 30g; Fiber 0.5g

43. Ginger Stir-Fry with Bok Choy and Peppers

Preparation time: Ten mins

Cooking time: Fifteen mins

Servings: Four

Ingredients:

- Two cups bok choy, chopped

- One cup red bell pepper, sliced into strips

- One tbsp grated fresh ginger

- Three tbsp soy sauce (gluten-free)

- Two tsp sesame oil

- Half-pound shrimp, peeled and deveined

- One-fourth cup green onions, sliced

Directions:

1. Warm up your big non-stick skillet on moderate-high temp and add sesame oil. Add ginger and stir-fry for one minute till fragrant.

2. Add shrimp, then cook for three mins per side till they turn pink. Remove the shrimp, then put aside.

3. In your same skillet, add bok choy and red bell pepper strips, then stir-fry for four to five mins till vegetables are tender.

4. Add shrimp and soy sauce over mixture, then toss well for one minute. Sprinkle green onions on top, then serve.

Serving Size: One cup stir-fry mixture with shrimp

Nutritional Values (per serving): Calories 150; Carbs 6g; Fat 4g; Protein 18g; Fiber 1g

44. Sheet Pan Za'atar Chicken with Sweet Potatoes

Preparation time: Fifteen mins

Cooking time: Thirty-five mins

Servings: Four

Ingredients:

- Four boneless, skinless chicken breasts

- One lb. sweet potatoes, peeled & cut into half-inch pieces

- Two tbsp olive oil

- Two tbsp za'atar seasoning

- One tsp garlic powder

- Half tsp sea salt

Directions:

1. Warm up your oven to 400°F. In your big container, toss sweet potatoes with one tbsp oil, quarter tsp sea salt, and half tbsp za'atar seasoning till coated. Spread them on one side of your sheet pan.

2. Rub chicken breasts with the remaining oil, za'atar seasoning, garlic powder, and sea salt. Put chicken on the other side of your sheet pan.

3. Bake for thirty-five mins till chicken is cooked through. Serve.

Serving Size: One chicken breast with quarter of the sweet potatoes.

Nutritional Values (per serving): Calories: 350; Carbs: 27g; Fat: 14g; Protein: 34g; Fiber: 4g

45. *Spinach & Mushroom Quinoa Risotto*

Preparation time: Ten mins

Cooking time: Twenty mins

Servings: Four

Ingredients:

- One cup quinoa, washed

- Two cups vegetable broth

- One lb. white mushrooms, sliced

- Three cups baby spinach leaves

- One tbsp olive oil

- One tsp thyme leaves

- Half tsp sea salt

Directions:

1. Warm up oil in your big pan on moderate temp. Add mushrooms, then cook for five mins till they start to release their juices.

2. Mix in quinoa and thyme leaves, then cook for another two mins. Pour in broth, then let it simmer.

3. Cover, adjust to low temp, then cook for fifteen mins till quinoa is tender. Remove, then mix in spinach leaves till wilted. Flavor it using sea salt, then serve.

Serving Size: One quarter of the entire dish

Nutritional Values (per serving): Calories: 260; Carbs: 39g; Fat: 8g; Protein: 11g; Fiber: 6g

46. Ginger Miso Soup with Noodles and Greens

Preparation time: Fifteen mins

Cooking time: Twenty mins

Servings: Four

Ingredients:

- Four cups vegetable broth
- One cup sliced mushrooms
- Two tbsp miso paste
- One tsp grated ginger
- Two cups cooked soba noodles
- Four cups chopped kale or spinach
- One tbsp olive oil

Directions:

1. In a big pot, warm up oil on moderate temp. Add mushrooms and ginger, then sauté for three mins. Pour broth, then let it simmer.

2. Put miso paste in your small container, add some hot broth, and whisk till smooth. Add it back into your pot.

3. Add the cooked soba noodles and greens, then let them warm through for five mins, ensuring not to boil to keep the benefits of miso intact. Serve hot.

Serving Size: One and a half cups

Nutritional Values (per serving): Calories: 260; Carbs: 35g; Fat: 8g; Protein: 12g; Fiber: 4g

47. *Turmeric & Ginger Chicken Soup*

Preparation time: Twenty mins

Cooking time: Thirty mins

Servings: Four

Ingredients:

- Two lbs. chicken breast, cut into chunks
- Four cups chicken broth
- One cup diced carrots
- One tsp turmeric powder
- One tsp freshly grated ginger
- Half cup coconut milk

Directions:

1. Put chicken chunks in your big pot and cover with broth. Add turmeric powder and ginger.
2. Let it boil on high temp, adjust to moderate-low temp and simmer for twenty-five mins till chicken is cooked through. Add carrots during the last ten mins of cooking.
3. Mix in coconut milk and simmer for five mins. Serve.

Serving Size: One and a half cups

Nutritional Values (per serving): Calories: 310; Carbs: 8g; Fat: 13g; Protein: 39g; Fiber: 2g

48. *Baked Pesto Halibut with Cherry Tomatoes*

Preparation time: Fifteen mins

Cooking time: Twenty mins

Servings: Four

Ingredients:

- Four (six-ounce) pieces of halibut fillets

- Two tbsp pesto sauce (store bought or homemade without cheese)

- One cup cherry tomatoes, halved

- One tbsp extra virgin olive oil

- One tsp garlic, minced

- Half tsp sea salt

- Quarter tsp black pepper

Directions:

1. Warm up your oven to 375°F. In your baking dish, put halibut fillets skin-side down. Spread half a tbsp pesto onto each fillet.

2. Scatter the cherry tomatoes around your fish. Drizzle oil and sprinkle with garlic, sea salt, and pepper on top.

3. Bake for twenty mins till the fish flakes easily. Serve.

Serving Size: One piece of halibut with tomatoes.

Nutritional Values (per serving): Calories 295; Carbs 6g; Fat 15g; Protein 34g; Fiber 2g

49. Baked Eggplant and Zucchini Casserole

Preparation time: Twenty mins

Cooking time: Thirty-five mins

Servings: Four

Ingredients:

- Three cups eggplant, diced into one-inch pieces

- Two cups zucchini, sliced into half-inch rounds

- Two tbsp olive oil

- One tbsp balsamic vinegar

- One cup natural tomato sauce (no sugar added)

- One tsp dried oregano

- Half tsp sea salt

Directions:

1. Warm up your oven to 400°F. Toss eggplant, zucchini, oil, balsamic vinegar, oregano, and sea salt in your big container till well coated.

2. Spread them in an even layer in your big baking dish. Pour tomato sauce on top. Cover using foil and bake for thirty-five mins till vegetables are tender.

Serving Size: Quarter of the casserole

Nutritional Values (per serving): Calories 160; Carbs 19g; Fat 9g; Protein 4g; Fiber 6g

50. Coconut Curry Tofu with Broccoli Florets

Preparation time: fifteen mins

Cooking time: twenty mins

Servings: Four

Ingredients:

- One lb. of firm tofu, pressed and cubed

- Two tbsp of olive oil

- Three cups of broccoli florets

- One can (fourteen oz) of coconut milk

- Two tbsp of curry powder

- One tsp salt

- Half cup vegetable broth

Directions:

1. In your big skillet, warm up oil on moderate temp and add tofu cubes. Cook tofu for ten mins till golden brown.

2. Add broccoli florets, then sauté for five mins. Pour coconut milk and broth, then mix in curry powder and salt.

3. Let it boil, then simmer for ten mins till broccoli is tender. Serve.

Serving Size: One-fourth of total dish

Nutritional Values (per serving): Calories 450; Carbs 18g; Fat 29g; Protein 22g; Fiber 5g

Quick Snacks and Small Bites

51. Turmeric Spiced Roasted Nuts

Preparation time: Five mins

Cooking time: twenty mins

Servings: Four

Ingredients:

- One cup raw mixed nuts
- One tbsp olive oil
- One tsp ground turmeric
- Half tsp garlic powder
- Half tsp ground cumin
- Quarter tsp sea salt
- One-eighth tsp black pepper

Directions:

1. Warm up your oven to 350°F. In your container, mix oil with turmeric, garlic powder, cumin, salt, and pepper. Add nuts, then toss well.

2. Spread the nuts on your lined baking sheet. Roast for twenty mins till golden brown, mixing halfway through. Cool it down, then serve.

Serving Size: Quarter cup

Nutritional Values (per serving): Calories: 204; Carbs: 9g; Fat: 18g; Protein: 5g; Fiber: 3g

52. Ginger Infused Pear Slices

Preparation time: Ten mins

Cooking time: N/A

Servings: Four

Ingredients:

- Four ripe pears, cored and sliced

- Two tbsp lemon juice

- One tbsp freshly grated ginger root

- Half tsp ground cinnamon

- One-eighth tsp ground nutmeg

Directions:

1. In your big container, whisk lemon juice, ginger, cinnamon, and nutmeg.

2. Add the pear slices to the bowl and gently toss them with the ginger infusion till well covered. Serve.

Serving Size: One pear

Nutritional Values (per serving): Calories: 95; Carbs: 25g; Fat: 0.2g; Protein: 0.6g; Fiber: 5.1g

53. Omega-3 Rich Avocado Dip with Crackers

Preparation time: fifteen mins

Cooking time: N/A

Servings: Four

Ingredients:

- Three medium ripe avocados

- Two tbsp fresh lime juice

- One tsp garlic powder

- Half tsp cayenne pepper

- Quarter cup chopped cilantro

- Salt to taste

- Your choice of gluten-free crackers for serving

Directions:

1. Peel and pit the avocados, then mash them in a medium bowl. Add the lime juice, garlic powder, cayenne pepper, and cilantro. Mix well, then season with salt.

2. Serve immediately with crackers.

Serving Size: Quarter of the dip and a handful of crackers

Nutritional Values (per serving): Calories: 204; Carbs: 17g; Fat: 15g; Protein: 2g; Fiber: 7g

54. *Sweet Potato and Kale Chips*

Preparation time: Ten mins

Cooking time: Twenty-five mins

Servings: Four

Ingredients:

- Two big sweet potatoes, thinly sliced

- One big bunch of kale, torn into bite-size pieces

- Three tbsp extra-virgin olive oil

- One tsp smoked paprika

- Half tsp sea salt

- Quarter tsp black pepper

Directions:

1. Warm up your oven to 350°F. Toss sweet potatoes and kale pieces with oil till coated.

2. Sprinkle paprika, sea salt, and black pepper over them, then toss again. Spread the sweet potato slices and kale pieces on your lined baking sheets.

3. Bake for twenty to twenty-five mins till crispy, turning halfway through.

Serving Size: One cup mixed sweet potato and kale chips

Nutritional Values (per serving): Calories: 207; Carbs: 23g; Fat: 12g; Protein: 3g; Fiber: 4g

55. Chickpea Hummus with Veggie Sticks

Preparation time: Five mins

Cooking time: N/A

Servings: Four

Ingredients:

- Two cups canned chickpeas, strained & washed
- Three tbsp of extra virgin olive oil
- One tbsp tahini
- Two tbsp of fresh lemon juice
- One tsp of minced garlic
- Half tsp of salt
- Assorted veggie sticks (cucumber, carrot, bell pepper)

Directions:

1. Combine chickpeas, olive oil, tahini, lemon juice, garlic, and salt in a food processor or blender.
2. Blend till smooth. Serve with an assortment of veggie sticks.

Serving Size: One-fourth of the total quantity

Nutritional Values (per serving): Calories 210; Carbs 20g; Fat 12g; Protein 7g; Fiber 6g

56. Grilled Pineapple with Cinnamon Drizzle

Preparation time: Ten mins

Cooking time: Eight mins

Servings: Four

Ingredients:

- One medium-sized pineapple, peeled, cored & cut into eight rings
- One tbsp honey

- Half tsp ground cinnamon

- One tbsp fresh lime juice

- One tsp coconut oil for grilling

- A pinch of salt

Directions:

1. Warm up your grill to medium-high heat and brush with coconut oil. In your small container, combine honey, cinnamon, lime juice, and salt.

2. Grill pineapple rings for three to four mins per side till they have nice grill marks. Drizzle the cinnamon mixture over the warm pineapple before serving.

Serving Size: Two pineapple rings with drizzle

Nutritional Values (per serving): Calories 100; Carbs 25g; Fat 1g; Protein 1g; Fiber 2g

57. Almond Butter & Banana Rice Cakes

Preparation time: Five mins

Cooking time: N/A

Servings: Four

Ingredients:

- Four rice cakes

- Four tbsp almond butter

- Two medium bananas

- One tsp chia seeds

- One tsp honey (optional)

- One pinch of cinnamon (optional)

Directions:

1. Spread one tbsp almond butter evenly over each rice cake. Slice the bananas thinly, then place the slices on top of the almond butter on each rice cake.

2. Sprinkle quarter tsp of chia seeds over each rice cake. If desired, drizzle quarter tsp of honey and cinnamon for added flavor. Serve.

Serving Size: One rice cake with toppings

Nutritional Values (per serving): Calories 210; Carbs 27g; Fat 11g; Protein 5g; Fiber 4g

58. Cherry Tomato & Basil Bruschetta

Preparation time: Ten mins

Cooking time: Five mins

Servings: Four

Ingredients:

- Eight slices whole-grain baguette
- Two cups cherry tomatoes, halved
- Four tbsp chopped fresh basil
- Two tsp extra virgin olive oil
- Half tsp balsamic vinegar
- One clove garlic, minced
- Salt and pepper to taste

Directions:

1. Warm up your broiler to high and place baguette slices on a baking sheet. Broil for one to two mins till just golden brown. Keep an eye on them to avoid burning.
2. In your container, combine cherry tomatoes, chopped basil, olive oil, balsamic vinegar, and minced garlic.
3. Season with salt and pepper and toss gently to mix. Spoon the tomato mixture evenly atop the toasted baguette slices. Serve while the bread is still warm and crisp.

Serving Size: Two bruschetta slices

Nutritional Values (per serving): Calories 150; Carbs 18g; Fat 6g; Protein 4g; Fiber 3g

59. Walnut Stuffed Dates with Honey Glaze

Preparation time: Five mins

Cooking time: N/A

Servings: Four

Ingredients:

- Sixteen whole pitted dates
- Eight tsp chopped walnuts
- Four tbsp honey, preferably raw
- One tsp ground cinnamon
- One tsp extra virgin olive oil
- A pinch of sea salt

Directions:

1. In your small container, mix the chopped walnuts with ground cinnamon and sea salt. Stuff each date with half tsp of the walnut mixture.

2. Drizzle the stuffed dates with honey. Lightly brush a serving platter with olive oil and arrange the dates on it.

Serving Size: Four stuffed dates

Nutritional Values (per serving): Calories: 230; Carbs: 35g; Fat: 10g; Protein: 2g; Fiber: 3g

60. Pumpkin Seeds and Goji Berry Trail Mix

Preparation time: Ten mins

Cooking time: N/A

Servings: Four

Ingredients:

- Half cup raw pumpkin seed (pepitas)
- Half cup goji berries, dried

- Quarter cup shelled sunflower seeds, raw

- Four tsp chia seeds

- Two tbsp unsweetened coconut flakes

- Quarter tsp ground turmeric

- One pinch ground black pepper

Directions:

1. In your big container, combine pumpkin seeds, goji berries, sunflower seeds, chia seeds, coconut flakes, turmeric, and black pepper.

2. Toss well to ensure all ingredients are mixed thoroughly. Portion the trail mix into individual servings or store in an airtight container.

Serving Size: Quarter cup

Nutritional Values (per serving): Calories: 180; Carbs: 20g; Fat: 10g; Protein: 6g; Fiber: 4g

Healthy Desserts

61. Refreshing Ginger Peach Sorbet

Preparation time: Fifteen mins

Cooking time: N/A

Servings: Four

Ingredients:

- Four ripe peaches, peeled and diced

- Quarter cup honey

- One tbsp fresh ginger, minced

- The juice of one lemon

- Two tbsp of water

Directions:

1. Blend the peaches, honey, ginger, and lemon juice with water till smooth. Transfer the mixture into a shallow dish and freeze for four hours, scraping with a fork every hour.

2. Once frozen, whisk to create a smooth sorbet texture and serve immediately or freeze till serving.

Serving Size: Half cup

Nutritional Values (per serving): Calories 104; Carbs 8g; Fat 1g; Protein 1g; Fiber 4g

62. Turmeric Spiced Almond Cookies

Preparation time: Ten mins

Cooking time: Twelve mins

Servings: Eight

Ingredients:

- One cup almond flour

- Three tbsp coconut oil, melted

- Three tbsp maple syrup

- One tsp ground turmeric

- Half tsp ground ginger

- Quarter tsp sea salt

- One tsp vanilla extract

Directions:

1. Warm up your oven to 350°F. Mix all ingredients in your container till well combined.

2. Scoop dough onto a baking sheet lined with parchment paper, pressing each cookie flat. Bake for twelve mins till edges are golden brown.

3. Cool on the baking sheet before transferring to a wire rack to cool completely.

Serving Size: One cookie

Nutritional Values (per serving): Calories 214; Carbs 8g; Fat 4g; Protein 1g; Fiber 2g

63. Golden Milk Frozen Yogurt Bark

Preparation time: Fifteen mins

Cooking time: N/A

Servings: Eight

Ingredients:

- Two cups plain Greek yogurt

- One tbsp turmeric

- Two tbsp honey

- One tsp ground cinnamon

- One tsp vanilla extract

- A pinch of black pepper

Directions:

1. In your container, mix Greek yogurt with turmeric, honey, cinnamon, vanilla extract, and black pepper.

2. Spread the mixture evenly on a lined baking sheet. Freeze for at least four hours till firm.

3. Break into pieces and serve immediately or store in an airtight container in the freezer.

Serving Size: One piece

Nutritional Values (per serving): Calories 90; Carbs 11g; Fat 2g; Protein 10g; Fiber 0.5g

64. Cherry Ginger Compote over Cashew Cream

Preparation time: Ten mins

Cooking time: Ten mins

Servings: Four

Ingredients:

- Two cups of fresh cherries, pitted and halved

- One tbsp freshly grated ginger

- Three tbsp of water

- One tbsp pure maple syrup

- One cup raw cashews, soaked overnight and drained

- One tsp of lemon juice

- A pinch of sea salt

Directions:

1. Blend cashews with lemon juice, sea salt, and two tbsp of water till smooth to make the cream.

2. Simmer cherries with grated ginger and the remaining tbsp water in a saucepan on moderate temp for ten mins till soft.

3. Stir in maple syrup and cook for an additional two mins. Let the compote cool slightly before serving over the cashew cream.

Serving Size: Half cup

Nutritional Values (per serving): Calories 200; Carbs 24g; Fat 11g; Protein 5g; Fiber 3g

65. *Pineapple Cilantro Lime Sorbet*

Preparation time: Ten mins

Cooking time: N/A

Servings: Four

Ingredients:

- Two cups fresh pineapple, diced
- One tbsp fresh lime juice
- One tbsp finely chopped cilantro
- Quarter cup honey (make sure it's pure honey with no additives)
- Quarter tsp sea salt

Directions:

1. Combine the pineapple, lime juice, cilantro, honey, and sea salt in a blender. Blend till completely smooth. Pour the mixture into a shallow container.

2. Cover and freeze till firm, usually around four to five hours, mixing it every hour if possible to add air into the sorbet and break up ice crystals.

3. Once frozen, let it sit at room temperature for five to ten mins before serving.

Serving Size: Half cup

Nutritional Values (per serving): Calories 120; Carbs 31g; Fat 0g; Protein 0g; Fiber 2g

66. *Baked Pears with Walnuts and Honey*

Preparation time: Ten mins

Cooking time: Twenty-five mins

Servings: Four

Ingredients:

- Four ripe but firm pears, halved and cored

- Four tsp raw honey

- Eight halves walnuts, crushed

- One tsp ground cinnamon

Directions:

1. Warm up your oven to 350°F. Place the pear halves cut-side up on a baking dish. Drizzle each pear half with half tsp of honey, then sprinkle with cinnamon.

2. Place a walnut half on top of each pear. Bake for twenty-five mins till the pears are tender and golden. Serve.

Serving Size: one half pear

Nutritional Values (per serving): Calories 150; Carbs 27g; Fat 3g; Protein 1g; Fiber 5g

67. Dark Chocolate Berry Cups

Preparation time: Ten mins

Cooking time: N/A

Servings: Four

Ingredients:

- Two-thirds cup dark chocolate chips (at least 70% cacao)

- One cup mixed berries

- Two tbsp of almond butter

- Two tsp chia seeds

- One tsp vanilla extract

- A pinch of sea salt

Directions:

1. Melt the dark chocolate chips using a double boiler method or microwave in thirty-second intervals, stirring till smooth.

2. Mix in the almond butter, vanilla extract, and sea salt with the melted chocolate. Place paper liners in a mini muffin tin. Pour two tsp of the chocolate mixture into each liner.

3. Add a spoonful of mixed berries into each cup and sprinkle chia seeds on top. Place in the freezer for at least one hour till set. Enjoy chilled.

Serving Size: One berry cup

Nutritional Values (per serving): Calories: 180; Carbs: 12g; Fat: 11g; Protein: 4g; Fiber: 3g

68. Mango Coconut Gelato

Preparation time: Fifteen mins

Cooking time: N/A

Servings: Four

Ingredients:

- Two cups of frozen mango chunks
- One-half cup full-fat coconut milk
- Two tbsp of honey or maple syrup (optional)
- One tbsp lime juice
- One tsp lime zest
- A pinch of sea salt

Directions:

1. Place frozen mango chunks into a food processor or high-powered blender. Add coconut milk, honey or maple syrup if using, lime juice, lime zest, and sea salt.
2. Blend till smooth and creamy, scraping down sides as necessary.
3. Serve immediately for a softer texture or transfer to an airtight container and freeze for two hours for a firmer consistency.

Serving Size: Half a cup

Nutritional Values (per serving): Calories: 150; Carbs: 25g; Fat: 6g; Protein: 1g; Fiber: 2g

69. Honey Drizzled Berries with Mint

Preparation time: Five mins

Cooking time: N/A

Servings: Two

Ingredients:

- Two cups mixed berries (blueberries, raspberries, strawberries)
- One tbsp raw honey
- One tbsp fresh mint leaves, finely chopped
- Half tsp freshly squeezed lemon juice

Directions:

1. Rinse the mixed berries and place them into two serving bowls. Drizzle one tbsp raw honey evenly over the berries in each bowl.
2. Sprinkle the finely chopped mint leaves on top of the honeyed berries. Finish by adding a splash of lemon juice to each serving for an added zing.

Serving Size: One cup

Nutritional Values (per serving): Calories 150; Carbs 37g; Fat 0.5g; Protein 2g; Fiber 6g

70. Coconut Ginger Rice Pudding

Preparation time: Five mins

Cooking time: Twenty-five mins

Servings: Four

Ingredients:

- One cup basmati rice, rinsed and drained
- Two cups canned coconut milk
- Two tbsp grated fresh ginger
- Three tbsp raw honey
- One tsp ground cinnamon
- Quarter cup raisins (optional)

- Pinch of salt

Directions:

1. In a medium-sized pot, mix basmati rice and coconut milk. Stir in the ginger, salt, and ground cinnamon.

2. Let it boil on moderate-high temp, then adjust to low heat. Cover and let simmer for twenty-five mins till the rice is tender.

3. Remove and stir in the raw honey and raisins if you're using them. Allow to cool slightly before serving warm, or chill in the refrigerator if preferred cold.

Serving Size: Three-quarters of a cup

Nutritional Values (per serving): Calories 260; Carbs 38g; Fat 12g; Protein 3g; Fiber 1g

71. Cinnamon Baked Apples

Preparation time: Ten mins

Cooking time: Twenty-five mins

Servings: Four

Ingredients:

- Four big apples, cored and sliced

- Two tbsp extra virgin olive oil

- One tbsp ground cinnamon

- One tsp vanilla extract

- Quarter cup chopped walnuts

- Two tbsp honey (optional, for sweetness)

- A pinch of salt

Directions:

1. Warm up your oven to 350°F. In your big container, toss the sliced apples with olive oil, cinnamon, vanilla extract, and a pinch of salt.

2. Transfer the apple mixture to a baking dish and sprinkle with chopped walnuts. Drizzle honey over the top if desired for added sweetness.

3. Bake for twenty-five mins till apples are tender. Serve warm.

Serving Size: One-fourth of total dish

Nutritional Values (per serving): Calories: 210; Carbs: 34g; Fat: 10g; Protein: 2g; Fiber: 5g

72. Easy Sweet Potato Brownies

Preparation time: Fifteen mins

Cooking time: Thirty mins

Servings: Eight

Ingredients:

- One big sweet potato (one lb.), peeled and mashed

- One-half cup almond flour

- Two tbsp unsweetened cocoa powder

- Three tbsp coconut oil

- Quarter cup pure maple syrup

- One tsp baking powder

- A pinch of salt

Directions:

1. Warm up your oven to 350°F. Grease an eight-inch square baking pan with a little coconut oil.

2. In your big container, mix together the sweet potato, almond flour, cocoa powder, coconut oil, maple syrup, baking powder, and salt till well combined.

3. Spread the batter evenly in your baking pan. Bake for thirty mins till an inserted toothpick comes out clean. Allow the brownies to cool before slicing into pieces.

Serving Size: One-eighth of total dish

Nutritional Values (per serving): Calories: 180; Carbs: 21g; Fat: 9g; Protein: 3g; Fiber: 4g

73. *Zesty Lemon Olive Oil Cake*

Preparation time: Fifteen mins

Cooking time: Thirty-five mins

Servings: Eight

Ingredients:

- Two cups of almond flour
- Half a cup olive oil
- Three-quarters of a cup honey
- Four tbsp of lemon juice
- Two tsp lemon zest
- One tsp baking soda
- One whole egg

Directions:

1. Warm up your oven to 325°F. In your container, combine the almond flour with baking soda.

2. In another container, whisk oil, honey, lemon juice, zest, and egg till well blended. Mix the wet ingredients into the dry ingredients till a smooth batter forms.

3. Pour batter into a greased nine-inch cake pan. Bake for thirty-five mins till a toothpick comes out clean. Cool before serving.

Serving Size: One slice

Nutritional Values (per serving): Calories: 315; Carbs: 23g; Fat: 24g; Protein: 5g; Fiber: 3g

74. *Matcha Green Tea Coconut Ice Cream*

Preparation time: Twenty mins + freezing time

Cooking time: N/A

Servings: Six

Ingredients:

- Two (14-oz) cans of full-fat coconut milk
- Quarter cup honey
- Four tbsp of matcha green tea powder
- One tsp vanilla extract

Directions:

1. Chill the coconut milk cans in the refrigerator overnight. The next day, scoop the firm coconut cream into your container, leaving any liquid behind.

2. Add honey and vanilla extract, then whisk vigorously till well combined. Sift matcha powder over the mixture and whisk till smooth and evenly distributed.

3. Pour mixture into a loaf pan or shallow dish and freeze for at least four hours till set. Let sit at room temperature for five mins to soften before scooping and serving.

Serving Size: One scoop

Nutritional Values (per serving): Calories: 300; Carbs: 20g; Fat: 25g; Protein: 2g; Fiber: 0g

75. Carrot Cake Oatmeal Cookies

Preparation time: Ten mins

Cooking time: Fifteen mins

Servings: Twelve

Ingredients:

- One cup rolled oats
- Two medium carrots, grated
- Quarter cup raw walnuts, chopped
- Quarter cup raisins
- Two tbsp coconut oil, melted
- Three tbsp pure maple syrup
- Half tsp ground cinnamon

Directions:

1. Warm up your oven to 350°F. In your big container, mix oats, carrots, walnuts, and raisins.

2. In a separate container, whisk coconut oil, maple syrup, and cinnamon till well combined. Combine wet and dry ingredients and stir till a dough forms.

3. Spoon tbsp-sized portions of the dough onto a baking sheet lined with parchment paper. Flatten each cookie slightly with the back of the spoon.

4. Bake for fifteen mins till cookies are lightly golden. Let the cookies cool on the baking sheet for five mins before transferring them to a wire rack to cool completely.

Serving Size: One cookie

Nutritional Values (per serving): Calories: 105; Carbs: 15g; Fat: 4g; Protein: 2g; Fiber: 2g

Drinks and Beverages

76. Turmeric Ginger Tea

Preparation time: Five mins

Cooking time: Ten mins

Servings: Two

Ingredients:

- Two cups water

- One tsp ground turmeric

- One tsp grated fresh ginger

- One tbsp honey

- Two tbsp lemon juice

- Pinch of black pepper

Directions:

1. In a small saucepan, bring water to a boil. Add ground turmeric and grated ginger to the boiling water.

2. Reduce heat and simmer for ten mins to allow the spices to infuse. Strain the tea into two cups then stir in honey, lemon juice, and black pepper. Serve warm.

Serving Size: One cup

Nutritional Values (per serving): Calories: 40; Carbs: 11g; Fat: 0g; Protein: 0g; Fiber: 0g

77. Pineapple Kale Smoothie

Preparation time: Five mins

Cooking time: N/A

Servings: Two

Ingredients:

- Two cups fresh pineapple chunks

- One cup chopped kale, stems removed

- One tbsp chia seeds

- Half tsp grated ginger

- One cup unsweetened almond milk

- One tbsp raw honey (optional)

Directions:

1. Combine the pineapple chunks, chopped kale, chia seeds, and grated ginger in a blender. Pour the almond milk over the top.

2. Blend on high speed till smooth and creamy. Taste and add honey if desired, then blend again to mix.

3. Divide the smoothie between two glasses and serve immediately.

Serving Size: One glass

Nutritional Values (per serving): Calories 95; Carbs 20g; Fat 1g; Protein 3g; Fiber 4g

78. Carrot Beetroot Juice

Preparation time: Five mins

Cooking time: N/A

Servings: Two

Ingredients:

- Four medium-sized carrots

- Two small beetroots

- One tbsp grated fresh ginger

- Two cups of cold water

- One tbsp lemon juice

- One tsp ground turmeric

- A pinch of black pepper (optional, to enhance absorption of turmeric)

Directions:

1. Wash and peel the carrots and beetroots. Roughly chop them into chunks. Add the carrots, beetroots, grated ginger, and cold water into a high-speed blender.

2. Blend on high till smooth for about one minute.

3. Strain using a fine mesh sieve or a cheesecloth over your big container to remove the pulp, pressing to extract the juice.

4. Stir in the lemon juice, ground turmeric, and black pepper. Serve.

Serving Size: One and a half cups

Nutritional Values (per serving): Calories: 95; Carbs: 22g; Fat: 0.3g; Protein: 2g; Fiber: 5g

79. Lemon Ginger Detox Drink

Preparation time: Five mins

Cooking time: N/A

Servings: One

Ingredients:

- One cup warm water

- Two tbsp lemon juice

- One tbsp grated ginger root

- Quarter tsp ground turmeric

- One tsp raw honey (optional)

- One pinch of cayenne pepper

Directions:

1. Warm one cup water to just below boiling. Add lemon juice and ginger root to a mug. Pour warm water into the mug and stir well.

2. Stir in ground turmeric, cayenne pepper, and raw honey if desired till well blended. Allow drink to steep for four mins then stir once more before drinking.

Serving Size: One cup

Nutritional Values (per serving): Calories: 11; Carbs: 3g; Fat: 0g; Protein: 0g; Fiber: 0g

80. Cherry Almond Milkshake

Preparation time: Five mins

Cooking time: N/A

Servings: Two

Ingredients:

- One cup unsweetened almond milk
- Two cups of frozen cherries
- One tbsp almond butter
- Half tsp vanilla extract
- One tbsp honey (optional)
- Ice cubes (optional)

Directions:

1. Combine the unsweetened almond milk, frozen cherries, almond butter, and vanilla extract in a blender.
2. Blend on high till smooth. If desired, add honey to sweeten and ice cubes for a thicker consistency.
3. Pour the milkshake into two glasses and serve immediately.

Serving Size: One cup

Nutritional Values (per serving): Calories 200; Carbs 30g; Fat 5g; Protein 2g; Fiber 3g

81. Refreshing Cucumber Mint Water

Preparation time: Ten mins

Cooking time: N/A

Servings: Four

Ingredients:

- Two medium cucumbers, thinly sliced

- Ten mint leaves

- Eight cups of water

- Ice cubes (optional)

Directions:

1. In a big pitcher, combine the sliced cucumbers and mint leaves. Fill the pitcher with water and stir gently.

2. Refrigerate for at least one hour to allow the flavors to infuse. Serve in glasses with additional ice cubes if preferred.

Serving Size: Two cups

Nutritional Values (per serving): Calorie 0; Carbs 0g; Fat 0g; Protein 0g; Fiber 0g

82. Blueberry Spinach Shake

Preparation time: Five mins

Cooking time: N/A

Servings: Two

Ingredients:

- One cup fresh blueberries

- Two cups baby spinach leaves

- One tbsp ground flaxseed

- Half a banana

- One cup Greek yogurt, plain

- Three-quarters cup water or as needed for blending

- A pinch of cinnamon

Directions:

1. Place blueberries, spinach leaves, ground flaxseed, and banana in a blender. Add Greek yogurt and a pinch of cinnamon.

2. Pour in water for easier blending. Blend on high till the mixture is smooth.

3. Pour into glasses and serve immediately or refrigerate for later use.

Serving Size: One glass

Nutritional Values (per serving): Calories 120; Carbs 18g; Fat 3g; Protein 7g; Fiber 3g

83. Pomegranate Green Smoothie

Preparation time: Five mins

Cooking time: N/A

Servings: Two

Ingredients:

- One cup pomegranate seeds

- Two cups of spinach leaves

- One tbsp chia seeds

- Half a cup unsweetened almond milk

- One big banana

- Ice cubes (optional)

- One tbsp honey (optional)

Directions:

1. In a blender, combine the pomegranate seeds, spinach, chia seeds, almond milk, and banana. Blend on high till smooth.

2. Taste and add ice cubes for a colder smoothie or honey for sweetness if desired. Blend again till the desired consistency is reached.

Serving Size: One and a half cups

Nutritional Values (per serving): Calories: 180; Carbs: 30g; Fat: 3g; Protein: 4g; Fiber: 5g

84. Spinach Flaxseed Power Drink

Preparation time: Five mins

Cooking time: N/A

Servings: Two

Ingredients:

- Two cups of fresh spinach leaves

- One cup unsweetened almond milk

- One ripe banana

- Two tbsp flaxseeds

- One tbsp honey

- Half tsp ground cinnamon

- Ice cubes (optional)

Directions:

1. Combine spinach, almond milk, banana, flaxseeds, honey, and cinnamon in a blender.

2. Blend on high speed till smooth. Add ice cubes if desired and blend till frosty.

Serving Size: One cup

Nutritional Values (per serving): Calories 180; Carbs 29g; Fat 4.5g; Protein 5g; Fiber 6g

85. Watermelon Cucumber Cooler

Preparation time: Five mins

Cooking time: N/A

Servings: Two

Ingredients:

- Four cups of cubed watermelon

- One medium cucumber, peeled and thinly sliced

- Juice of one lemon

- Two tbsp of fresh mint leaves

- One tbsp raw honey (optional)

Directions:

1. In a blender, combine watermelon, cucumber slices, lemon juice, and mint leaves. Pulse till completely blended and smooth.

2. Taste and add honey if more sweetness is desired. Blend again briefly to mix. Serve chilled or over ice.

Serving Size: Two cups

Nutritional Values (per serving): Calories: 90; Carbs: 22g; Fat: 0.5g; Protein: 2g; Fiber: 1g

28-DAY MEAL PLAN

DAY	BREAKFAST	LUNCH	DINNER	DESSERT
1	Omega Boost Avocado Toast	Stuffed Bell Peppers with Spinach	Ginger-Turmeric Cauliflower Steaks	Refreshing Ginger Peach Sorbet
2	Spinach and Tomato Omelette	Grilled Vegetable Hummus Wrap	Coconut Curry Tofu with Broccoli Florets	Carrot Cake Oatmeal Cookies
3	Apple Cinnamon Overnight Oats	Butternut Squash and Turmeric Soup	Baked Eggplant and Zucchini Casserole	Matcha Green Tea Coconut Ice Cream
4	Anti-Oxidant Rich Buckwheat Pancakes	Beetroot and Carrot Detox Salad	Baked Pesto Halibut with Cherry Tomatoes	Zesty Lemon Olive Oil Cake
5	Cauliflower Rice Breakfast Bowl	Curried Chickpea Lettuce Wraps	Ginger Stir-Fry with Bok Choy and Peppers	Honey Drizzled Berries with Mint
6	Kale and Mushroom Frittata	Lemon Garlic Baked Cod with Asparagus	Turmeric & Ginger Chicken Soup	Easy Sweet Potato Brownies
7	Flaxseed and Walnut Porridge	Spicy Lentil and Turmeric Soup	Ginger Miso Soup with Noodles and Greens	Cinnamon Baked Apples
8	Broccoli and Bell Pepper Mini Quiche	Smoked Salmon and Avocado Wrap	Spinach & Mushroom Quinoa Risotto	Coconut Ginger Rice Pudding
9	Green Tea Infused Chia Pudding	Tomatoes and Bell Pepper Gazpacho	Sheet Pan Za'atar Chicken with Sweet Potatoes	Golden Milk Frozen Yogurt Bark
10	Sweet Potato & Red Onion Hash	Berry Walnut Baby Spinach Salad	Black Bean Quinoa Casserole	Mango Coconut Gelato

11	Quinoa & Almond Breakfast Bars	Quick Broccoli Almond Soup	Citrus-Herb Baked Cod Fillets	Dark Chocolate Berry Cups
12	Chia Seed & Mixed Berry Parfait	Turkey, Spinach, and Cucumber Wrap	Balsamic Grilled Tempeh with Veggies	Baked Pears with Walnuts and Honey
13	Blueberry Spinach Smoothie Bowl	Sweet Potato and Lentil Stew	Spicy Tomato-Basil Farro with Olives	Cherry Ginger Compote over Cashew Cream
14	Turmeric Ginger Oatmeal	Wild Salmon and Roasted Veggie Bowl	Garlicky Shrimp and Broccoli Rabe	Pineapple Cilantro Lime Sorbet
15	Anti-Inflammatory Granola Clusters	Turmeric-Ginger Grilled Chicken	Omega -Rich Salmon with Zucchini Ribbons	Turmeric Spiced Almond Cookies
16	Omega Boost Avocado Toast	Stuffed Bell Peppers with Spinach	Ginger-Turmeric Cauliflower Steaks	Refreshing Ginger Peach Sorbet
17	Spinach and Tomato Omelette	Grilled Vegetable Hummus Wrap	Coconut Curry Tofu with Broccoli Florets	Carrot Cake Oatmeal Cookies
18	Apple Cinnamon Overnight Oats	Butternut Squash and Turmeric Soup	Baked Eggplant and Zucchini Casserole	Matcha Green Tea Coconut Ice Cream
19	Anti-Oxidant Rich Buckwheat Pancakes	Beetroot and Carrot Detox Salad	Baked Pesto Halibut with Cherry Tomatoes	Zesty Lemon Olive Oil Cake
20	Cauliflower Rice Breakfast Bowl	Curried Chickpea Lettuce Wraps	Ginger Stir-Fry with Bok Choy and Peppers	Honey Drizzled Berries with Mint
21	Kale and Mushroom Frittata	Lemon Garlic Baked Cod with Asparagus	Turmeric & Ginger Chicken Soup	Easy Sweet Potato Brownies

22	Flaxseed and Walnut Porridge	Spicy Lentil and Turmeric Soup	Ginger Miso Soup with Noodles and Greens	Cinnamon Baked Apples
23	Broccoli and Bell Pepper Mini Quiche	Smoked Salmon and Avocado Wrap	Spinach & Mushroom Quinoa Risotto	Coconut Ginger Rice Pudding
24	Green Tea Infused Chia Pudding	Tomatoes and Bell Pepper Gazpacho	Sheet Pan Za'atar Chicken with Sweet Potatoes	Golden Milk Frozen Yogurt Bark
25	Sweet Potato & Red Onion Hash	Berry Walnut Baby Spinach Salad	Black Bean Quinoa Casserole	Mango Coconut Gelato
26	Quinoa & Almond Breakfast Bars	Quick Broccoli Almond Soup	Citrus-Herb Baked Cod Fillets	Dark Chocolate Berry Cups
27	Chia Seed & Mixed Berry Parfait	Turkey, Spinach, and Cucumber Wrap	Balsamic Grilled Tempeh with Veggies	Baked Pears with Walnuts and Honey
28	Blueberry Spinach Smoothie Bowl	Sweet Potato and Lentil Stew	Spicy Tomato-Basil Farro with Olives	Cherry Ginger Compote over Cashew Cream

RECIPE INDEX

Conclusion

You now hold the knowledge and inspiration to transform your meals into a force for health, vitality, and flavor. The power of anti-inflammatory eating is not just a transient trend but a profound insight into how our diet impacts every aspect of our wellbeing.

With the nutritional science, practical advice, and a myriad of delectable recipes at your fingertips, you have everything you need to transition to an anti-inflammatory lifestyle that doesn't sacrifice taste or satisfaction. Remember that each spoonful of *Omega Boost Avocado Toast*, each crunch of *Turmeric Spiced Almond Cookies*, and each sip of your *Turmeric Ginger Tea* is not just nourishment for your body but also peace for your cells.

But beyond the nutrients and the antioxidants, it's about adopting a mindset rooted in self-care and intentionality. You have learned how to discern which foods serve your health and which ones to leave on the store shelf. Dr. Sebi's alkaline approach, along with tips for smart shopping and meal planning, has opened the door to a way of eating that supports your body's natural defenses against inflammation.

Maintaining this lifestyle is about more than just what's on your plate—it's about making informed choices whether you're dining out or cooking at home, sustaining motivation even when it's tough, and bouncing back from setbacks with grace. As you continue on this path, allow yourself flexibility and patience. A holistic approach means occasional indulgences are not just allowed; they are part of the joy of eating! Your commitment to reducing inflammation through diet doesn't require perfection; it thrives on balance and consistency.

So where do you go from here? Apply what you've learned. Begin with simple swaps and gradually build up to more elaborate recipes as your skills and confidence grow. Get creative with substitutions based on what produce is seasonal and fresh in your locality. Share your culinary creations with friends and family because healthy habits bloom more fully when nurtured within a community.

Listen to your body. It will tell you what it needs if you pay close enough attention. The way we feel after meals is our most direct feedback loop—use it wisely. Finally, extend this compassion toward yourself outwards—teach others about the benefits of an anti-inflammatory diet. Share this cookbook; spread knowledge about nourishing food; be the ripple effect in your community.

Made in the USA
Middletown, DE
02 September 2024